Anything Is Everything

Everything Is Nothing

Nothing Is Everything

The Wisdom to Live
As If Everything Is A Miracle

STEPHEN LAU

DEDICATION

This book is dedicated to those who appreciate life and living, and who believe that life is still a miracle.

All the quotes from Lao Tzu are taken from the author's own book **TAO TE CHING in Plain English**.

CONTENTS

INTRODUCTION

Living in this material world is all about struggling and surviving. The good news is that it is a human race in which there are really no real winners and losers in the end. But no matter what, we all have to finish that race somehow, with no exception. Just do your very best, and let the Creator do the rest to help you finish your own race with grace and dignity. The wisdom of your body, your mind, and your spirit may awaken and rejuvenate you along the rest of your life journey.

Living is always a discovery process. Life is a journey of self-discovery—finding *who* you are, *why* you are here, *what* you really need, and *how* you may meet your basic needs, so that you, like every one else, can fulfill some of your life goals and purposes that are exclusively designed for you. But to do just that, you need profound human wisdom and spiritual wisdom to continue that journey as if everything is a miracle.

Albert Einstein once said: "There are only two ways to live your life. One is as if nothing is a miracle. The other is as if everything is a miracle."

Indeed, life is a miracle in itself. Being alive is a miracle. Having your breaths is already a miracle. Everything in life *is* a miracle.

To truly believe and appreciate the miracle of life, you need the wisdom to grasp the full meaning of *anything is everything*, *everything is nothing*, and *nothing is everything*—they may all ultimately lead to your self-awakening, without which you will continue to live as if nothing is a miracle.

I sincerely hope that you will enjoy reading this book and find it self-enlightening as you continue the rest of your own life journey to reach your final destination.

Stephen Lau

<u>ONE</u>

ANYTHING IS EVERYTHING

The Meanings and the Interpretations

What is meant by "anything is everything"? It may have different meanings and different interpretations to different individuals.

First of all, human perceptions are subjective and individualized: they are affected not only by the five senses, but also by the unique experiences of an individual, as well as by the indelible memories of those experiences retained in the mind of that individual. Therefore, what is important to *you* may not be as important to *others*, and vice-versa. For this reason, *anything* could be *everything* to you, but not to others.

<u>An illustration</u>

Near the end of 2016, a road rage occurred in Arkansas that ended in the tragic death of a 3-year-old child.

A woman, with her 3-year-old grandson sitting at the back of her car, stopped at a stop sign. A man in the car right behind honked her for not starting her car immediately, but the woman honked back; thus the road rage began with the man firing a gun shot at the back of the woman's car.

Stopping too long at a stop sign, or wanting to get

to a place on time might be *everything* to the man. Having the right to remain where she was might also be *everything* to the woman, so she naturally honked back.

Unfortunately, that anything-is-everything incident ended in tragedy—the death of the woman's three-year-old grandson being shot dead while sitting at the back of her car.

In real life, *anything* could be *everything* to real people—it all depends on their respective perspectives of *anything is everything*.

Another illustration

In 2012, a Chinese couple from Hong Kong filed a lawsuit against an education consultant in the United States for $2 million dollars, who promised that he could—but ultimately did not—get their two sons into Harvard University.

The couple had used "improper" but maybe still perfectly "legal" means to get their two sons into Harvard University.

Getting into an elite college or university may be *everything* to many students, including their parents. Some might even resort to doing *anything* in order to achieve that goal, which is *everything* to them.

A similar illustration

A pastor from Hong Kong was invited to give a sermon in China. A woman from the congregation asked the pastor if it was "right" to give money to get her son into an elite school in China. The pastor replied by saying: "Your son getting into that elite school would also imply depriving another child of that same opportunity you are seeking for your child."

A year later, the pastor met the same woman, who

told him that her son had got into that elite school but without using her *kwganxi* or connection. The pastor then said to her: "See, God is in control; if you would just let Him."

Now, what is *your* own take on "anything is everything"?

A Frog in a Well

In many ways, many of us are just like a frog in a well, looking up at the limited sky above, in that we see only *ourselves*, and no one else, and therefore anything *is* everything to us. In other words, we see only our own needs and desires that have to be fulfilled and gratified no matter how, but without seeing those in others.

Just like the man in the car rage who saw only his own need to get going, but without even considering *why* the woman might be stalling her car at the stop sign and not moving ahead right away.

Just like the Chinese couple who saw only their desire to get their two sons into Harvard University, but without considering that their "improper action" might also deprive the opportunity of two other students to get into Harvard University.

These two examples above also illustrate another basic but major human flaw—the "inflated" ego-self, which is focusing too much on "anything is everything" related to an individual's ego-self.

We are all created to be in this world for only one purpose: to be our *true* self. Conventional wisdom often tells us to find our role model, pursue our life goals based on that role model. Subconsciously, we may all begin to dream that we are that role model or someone else that we are not, instead of being who we are supposed to be. That is *how* we may all have created an ego for ourselves; worse, we may even believe that we have to somehow gratify our ego-self in order to feel happy and contented.

The truth of the matter is that we *all* have an ego, and that is why we *all*, without any exception, have experienced unhappiness to a certain extent at some points in our lives. Unfortunately, the human ego is also the underlying cause or the main source of all human miseries and sufferings. That is to say, the human ego is the human flaw responsible for most of the problems and troubles that we are all facing in our lives.

The reality is that we cannot get rid of our ego because it is our uniquely individual identity. Having said that, we can still somehow diminish its size, or at least not letting it get out of control and dominate us eventually. Remember, the *size* of your ego is directly proportionate to the *degree* of distortion of your thinking mind, creating the so-called "realities" in your mind, which often are biased and untrue.

Your ego is your *perceived* identity, which is neither a social security number nor just a face. Your identity is your *inner self* or your *self-worth* as a person that *you* perceive. Many people even strive to build their identities by manipulating *acceptance* and *attention* from others. Sadly, that usually does not work: your true identify should be based on how *you* perceive yourself, rather than on how you perceive what *others* may think of you. That is to say, your true identity should not be built upon your own inflated ego.

The bottom line: like a frog in a well, with only limited and imperfect vision and perception of the sky above, you may then unconsciously distort your thinking mind with your inflated ego.

For example, the Chinese couple with an inflated ego might have developed an *assumptive prediction* that their sons going to Harvard University would lead to an excellent higher education, a successful career, followed by a good marriage, and hence living happily ever after. But, in real life, nothing could be further from the truth.

To be the frog that jumps out of the well to see anything and everything totally *different*, you need *both* human wisdom and spiritual wisdom.

Human Wisdom and Spiritual Wisdom

Wisdom is the capability of the thinking mind to draw sufficient conclusions from insufficient premises. We never have sufficient data for anything and everything because we are all limited in our capability in acquiring our knowledge.

Wisdom is not quite the same as knowledge: knowledge is the acquisition of facts and information, while wisdom is the application of acquired knowledge to everyday life and living. For this reason, being knowledgeable does not necessarily imply being wise. Wisdom is *beyond* knowledge.

Human Wisdom

Socrates, the famous Greek philosopher, once said: "An unexamined life is not worth living."

Wisdom is examining life by frequently asking self-intuitive questions, as well as by finding answers to the questions asked about life and living. In real life, we must frequently ask ourselves many questions about anything and everything at all times.

Asking relevant questions is introspection, which is a continual process of self-reflection, without which there is no self-awareness and hence no personal growth and development. A static life is never a life well lived. So, asking self-intuitive questions is self-empowering wisdom—a life-skill tool necessary for the art of living well.

Why is that?

It is because the kind of questions you ask also determines the kind of life you are going to live. Your questions often trigger a set of mental answers, which may lead to actions or inactions, based on the choices you have made from the answers you have obtained. Remember, your life is always the sum of all the choices you make in the process of going through your life journey.

To make the right daily life choices, you need human wisdom, which is clarity of thinking, to know *who* you really are, *what* choices are available to you, and *why* you decide on those choices.

TAO Wisdom

TAO is the profound human wisdom of **Lao Tzu**, the ancient sage from China, more than 2,600 years ago, who was the author of the immortal classic ***Tao Te Ching*** on human wisdom. (See **Appendix A: Tao Te Ching**.)

Spiritual Wisdom

Empower your mind with human wisdom to see things as what they really are, instead of as what they are supposed to be or what you wish they were. Before that could happen, however, you must know your real self *first*, that is, who you really are, and not your ego-self.

True human wisdom is not easy to attain or come by, especially living in this material world, which is a toxic environment. Living in a toxic environment, the human body may easily become contaminated, and thus ultimately infesting the human mind as well, given that the human body and the human mind are somehow interconnected.

An infested human mind often leads to distorted thinking—and that is where spiritual wisdom may play a pivotal role by giving the mind guidance, instruction, and supervision.

Ask yourself this thinking question: Do I have a soul or spirit?

If you do not totally *live* in your body, you *do* have a soul or spirit. If you do not totally *focus* on self, you may then also have a glimpse of your soul or spirit.

The next thinking question to ask yourself: What is my soul or spirit?

If you believe in God, your soul is your spiritual *connection* and *communication* with Him in the form of your daily prayers, moments of self-awakening, and occasional divine guidance and inspiration.

If you do not have a specific religion, but still believe in the control of a Being greater than yourself, your soul or spirit is your *understanding* of the unexplainable control and the natural cycle of all things—that is, certain things in life are beyond human control, and certain things follow a natural cycle or order, such as the cycle of the four seasons, and that life is inevitably followed by death.

If you are a non-believer, but still a decent human being, your soul or spirit is your *conscience*, which intuitively tells you what is right and wrong, and not just merely following the law and order of your country.

Therefore, in several different ways, we may all have a soul or spirit of some sort, although some of us may separate ourselves from it, either consciously or unconsciously. The soul or spirit is like a shadow of ourselves: sometimes we see more of it, and other times we see less of it, but it is always part and parcel of us, following us wherever we go, whether we like it or not.

<u>The role of spiritual wisdom</u>

Your soul may provide you with spiritual wisdom. As opposed to materiality, spirituality is something invisible and immeasurable, but is forever present and lasting. It is like the wind—invisible and yet palpable. It provides guidance, direction, and understanding to the mind. Spirituality may also take the form of love, joy, and peace, and it is often expressed in human actions and behaviors.

Materiality, on the other hand, is always visible, measurable, but is forever transient. Humans need *both* spirituality and materiality: the former to understand self, and the latter to understand the world and the universe around self. Spirituality not only inspires the mind but also energizes the body—it is a body-mind-soul connection necessary for the miracle of life and living.

Remember, your whole being is composed of the physical, the mental, and the spiritual. Your body—the physical—is controlled by your mind—the mental—and supervised by your soul—the spiritual. In other words, your spirituality oversees your whole being. Nothing transforms you as much as changing from a mundane to a spiritual attitude toward all your everyday life problems. To be spiritual, you must, first of all, look *beyond* yourself—that is, looking at *others*, instead of just focusing on yourself, like a frog in a well.

Oneness with All Life

With both human wisdom and spiritual wisdom, you may see *anything is everything* not just for yourself but also for others as well. In other words, you may intuit the wisdom of oneness with all life, which is your interconnection with others, not just with those who are close to you, but also with those who are distant and unrelated to you. Life is all about anything and everything.

No man is an island

According to **John Donne**, the famous English poet, "no man is an island"; that is, every man is a piece of the continent, a part of the main. Therefore, we are *all* interconnected with, as well as inter-dependent on, one another in many different ways.

Connectedness

Oneness is the law of nature: what we do to others, we also do to ourselves, either consciously or unconsciously. It is the *unity* of all life—life is what we all have, and what empowers all of us, giving us the enlightening experiences and the holistic ways of living.

The **Bible** has repeatedly stated the significance of oneness of God's creation and salvation to all.

> In the beginning was the Word, and the Word was with God, and the Word was God.
> (**John** 1: 1)

> For in him all things were created: things in heaven and on earth, visible and invisible, whether thrones or powers or rulers or authorities; all things have been created through him and for him.
> (**Colossians** 1: 16)

> For we were all baptized by one Spirit so as to form one body—whether Jews or Gentiles, slave or free—and we were all

given the one Spirit to drink.
(**1 Corinthians** 12:13)

According to **Lao Tzu**, the ancient Chinese sage, one of the reasons why nature has continued to exist for thousands and thousands of years is that all forms of life in nature have their presence, which depends on one another for their co-existence. Just think about that: everything in nature does not exist just for itself, and that is *why* it can last forever.

Each and every being in the universe.
is an expression of the Creator.
We are all shaped and perfected by Him.
(Lao Tzu, *Tao Te Ching*, Chapter 51)

Blessed is he who has no ego-self.
He will be rewarded with humility to connect with the Creator.
(Lao Tzu, *Tao Te Ching*, Chapter 9)

So, always focus on *others*, instead of just on yourself all the time. Focusing on others also initiates your connection with the Creator, providing you with spiritual wisdom to guide you along the rest of your life journey.

According to **Buddha**, "Nothing ever exists entirely alone. Everything is in relation to everything else." What Buddha means is that it is not uncommon for humans to blame their problems on all the things *outside* themselves—other people and circumstances that are beyond their control. But the connectedness with all life contradicts that common but erroneous belief; the reality is that what we see in others and in our own circumstances is a reflection of our inner life, of what we believe in—which is the main source of all human miseries and sufferings. The truth is that all humans suffer because they do not see the miseries and sufferings in others, except in themselves.

Martin Luther King, Jr., Baptist minister, and leader in the civil rights movement, once said: "Whatever affects one directly, affects all indirectly. I can never be what I ought to be until you are what you ought to be. This is the interrelated structure of reality." So, your connectedness to others plays a pivotal role in helping you become your true self, instead of who you wish you were.

Even **John Lennon** in his famous hit song "Imagine" says: "You may say I'm a dreamer, but I'm not the only one. I hope one day you'll join us. And the world will live as one." That the world will live as one may indeed become a reality, and not just a dream.

So, oneness is focusing on *wholeness*, connecting anything and everything, not just in the world we are living in but also in the whole universe that is beyond us.

This once intricate and inexplicable connectedness is now no longer a religious, spiritual, or philosophical concept; it has become a clear scientific principle for further exploration and more investigation. Indeed, many celebrated quantum physicists, ecologists, and environmentalists have now come to believe that all life and matter are united by an underlying *energy* or *consciousness*.

This scientific belief is also a strong testament to what **Albert Einstein** had previously said: "A human being is a part of the whole called by us universe, a part limited in time and space. He experiences himself, his thoughts and feelings as something separated from the rest, a kind of optical delusion of his consciousness. This delusion is a kind of prison for us, restricting persons nearest to us. Our task must be to free ourselves from this prison by widening our circle of compassion to embrace all living creatures and the whole of nature in its beauty."

The bottom line: oneness with all life may lead to your diverse expressions of the one original source energy, and thus enabling you to grow spiritually toward your further understanding of the oneness with all life.

Love and Forgiveness

Love

"Love" is a big word in all human civilizations. For all religious disparities, love still plays an essential role in all the world's religions. Love plays an important role in human lives and happiness, especially living in a world of aggression and depression.

What is the real meaning of "love"? Love involves our emotions and feelings. We all love some things and some people. Love, ironically enough, gives us *both* happiness and unhappiness. When the love is fulfilled, we feel happy; when the love is rejected or unrequited, we then feel the pain, which becomes the unhappiness. That, unfortunately, is also the reality of love.

In Christianity, "love" refers to the love of God and the love of your neighbors or even your enemies. In Buddhism, love refers to an awakened state of mind; the word "Buddha" means "wake up."

If you want to love others—no matter whether they deserve your love or not—you must love yourself *first*, and that is also the reality of life and love. Ironically enough, it is not easy to love yourself, let alone loving others, especially those you are not particularly fond of.

The truth of the matter is that in our connection with others, while expressing the one original source energy of love, we may see ourselves better than others, or others are better than ourselves. In the former situation, with a greater ego, we may demand others to gratify ourselves *first* before expressing our love to them; in the latter situation, with lower self-esteem, we may become hesitant in loving others as we should, thinking that our love may be rejected due to our perception of our own unworthiness.

No matter what your perception of self may be, always focus on your *connectedness* to others, instead of just focusing on yourself, especially your own ego-self. According to **Oslo**, a charismatic spiritual leader of India, "Love is happy when it is able to give something. Ego is happy when it is able to take something."

Remember, every person has a heart, and every heart has a place to love and to be loved, as well as to be connected to other hearts.

Always avail yourself of every opportunity in life to express your love and care to others. You pass through life only once, so show your love *now*, and not later.

Self-acceptance

To *truly* love someone is very difficult, if not impossible, unless you love yourself *first*, which is self-acceptance—accepting who and what you really are, and not who and what you wish you were (which is your ego-self). It should also be pointed out that "loving yourself" and "loving your ego-self" are not quite the same. The former is about loving yourself for who you really are despite all your imperfections; the latter is about craving to be the person you wish you were.

"Loving yourself" means you *can* also love others just as well because they are not very different from you in that they, too, are as imperfect as you are. On the other hand, "loving your ego-self" means it is very difficult to love others because you want to distinguish and separate yourself from others; accordingly, others must somehow satisfy your ego *first* before you can love them. That explains why if you have a big ego-self, you cannot easily and readily love others.

The bottom line: if you can accept yourself as who and what you are, then it may become much easier for you to accept and love others as who and what they are because you are not *different* or *separate* from others.

> The greatest virtue of all is to be unaware of a separate self at all.
> Awareness of a separate self makes us want to become valuable.
> Not becoming valuable, we tend to hate the separate self.
> Hating the separate self, how can we value anyone else?
>
> Freedom from the ego-self, we are free to act without the desire to be valuable.
> As a result, everything is done, and people all say: "It happened *naturally*."
> (Lao Tzu, **Tao Te Ching**, Chapter 17)

Forgiveness

Forgiveness is letting go of grudges and bitterness when you are hurt by someone. Forgiving is neither forgetting nor excusing the harm done to you. Instead of holding on to your anger, resentment, and thoughts of revenge, you now decide to embrace forgiveness and then move forward. In reality, you are actually embracing peace, hope, gratitude and joy—

the fundamentals of human happiness.

Forgiveness can also lead to the understanding of empathy and compassion for the one who hurt you. Forgiveness is a pathway to spirituality, and ultimately to human happiness.

<u>An illustration</u>

In September 24, 2016, runner and cyclist **Dean Otto** was struck by a car driven by **Will Huffman**, a 27-year-old salesman, with his buddy on their way to a football game. The crash left Dean Otto paralysed with his broken vertebrae, a broken pelvis, broken tailbone, a broken right leg, and several broken ribs.

After assessing Otto's condition, **Dr. Matt McGirt** told the Otto family that Dean Otto was 99 percent likely going to spend the rest of his days in a wheelchair. It was sad and scary news for the Otto family.

But Otto was never scared—or even resentful. Instead, he said a private prayer and instantly forgave Will Huffman. "I knew if I didn't, the resentment would eat me alive."

After the surgery on his spine performed by Dr. Matt McGirt, Otto began his miraculous recovery. As a matter of fact, a few hours after the surgery, Otto was able to wiggle his toes.

Through *Facebook*, Will Huffman and his wife were finally able to contact Otto's family, who welcomed them graciously with open arms.

Huffman was not surprised that Otto would forgive him, but he did not expect or imagine that they would become good friends afterwards. Huffman says, "I think most people would stop there and say, 'Nice meeting you, but I'm done.'"

Dr. Matt McGirt was also inspired by their close friendship, and he earnestly believed that it was Otto's attitude, forgiveness, and loving-kindness that had brought about his phenomenal recovery. The doctor also remarks: "He not only turned lemons into lemonade, but he's selling that lemonade, too." Otto raised $11,000 for Carolinas Rehabilitation's LIFE Program for spinal cord injury patients.

On July 22, 2017, Otto, Huffman, and Dr. McGirt reunited and participated in a half-marathon race.

Self-intuitive questions

- If I were Dean Otto, would I have forgiven Will Huffman instantly?

- Would I have continued the friendship with someone who drastically changed my life?

- Has forgiveness really made Dean Otto happier?

Spiritual wisdom

We must always forgive people their wrongs against us no matter how great the offense because God offers His forgiveness regardless of our own offenses. Therefore, we are expected to do the same, if we wish to receive His wisdom.

> Do not judge, and you will not be judged.
> Do not condemn, and you will not be condemned. Forgive, and you will be forgiven.
> (**Luke 6**: 37)

Conventional wisdom

According to the *Journal of Happiness Studies*, human happiness may come from the quality of the friendship or relationship experiences that promote the feeling of *uniqueness* in an individual.

<u>TAO Wisdom</u>

According to **Lao Tzu**, judging nothing, you will be happy; forgiving anything and everything, you will be happier; and loving anything and everything, you will be happiest. Not judging everyone you encounter gives you better understanding of humanity, and thus instrumental in learning new ways to love and to help others. Forgiveness is a powerful spiritual medicine that cures all negative emotions and feelings.

> The Creator seems elusive amid the changes of life.
> At times, He seems to have forsaken His creations.
> In reality, He is simply observing the comings and goings of their follies.
>
> Likewise, we watch the comings and goings
> of our likes and dislikes, of our desires and fears.
> But we do not identify with them.
> With no judgment and no preference,
> we see the mysteries of creation.
> (Lao Tzu, ***Tao Te Ching***, Chapter 7)
>
> Stop striving to be righteous and wise to attain salvation,
> which comes not from our efforts, not from something we must earn.
>
> Stop abiding by rules and regulations to secure fairness and justice.

Compassion and loving-kindness come naturally to us.
(Lao Tzu, ***Tao Te Ching***, Chapter 19)

True love is generosity, which is giving without expecting anything in return—a practical expression of compassion that provides lasting happiness and divine inspiration.

The Way may seem insignificant.
It is because it appears ordinary.
The Way is great beyond comparison.
If there were any comparison,
it would no longer be great.

The Way is great because of its three essentials:
compassion, humility, and faith.
With compassion, there is no fear.
With humility, there is no strife.
With faith, there is no impossibility.

Without compassion, fearlessness then becomes ruthlessness.
Without humility, efforts may become complicated and difficult.
Without faith, possibilities may become controlling and self-centering.
Compassion is the root.
Humility is the stem.
Faith is the flower.
(Lao Tzu, ***Tao Te Ching***, Chapter 67)

Gratitude and Generosity

Gratitude

Reconnect your soul or spirit to gratitude. If you are grateful to the Creator for what you have, you may look at the behavior of another individual with more tolerance, or even with a totally different perspective.

Blessings in life, such as the gift of life, are generally overlooked or even taken for granted. For example, if someone takes advantage of you, do not become angry immediately; instead, be grateful that you are the victim instead of being the person who victimizes others.

Gratitude enables you to develop the mindset for a positive outlook toward your soul. Smile more often. Keep complaints about people, things, and life in general only to *yourself*—unless voicing them will help bring about positive changes in others or in society.

Gratitude helps you see the good in others, letting you give them the benefit of the doubt. Try to remember that all people are created in the image of God. Focus on the individual as a person, rather than on the behavior or belief of that individual, which may not be appealing or pleasing to you.

Always be grateful that you have been given the opportunity to become either a teacher or a student in whatever circumstance you may find yourself in, and turn it into a miracle of life.

An illustration

At the end of 2007, **John Kralik**, an attorney who owned a law firm, experienced debts and disasters in both his life and his career.

One day, after a walk in the mountains, Kralik became enlightened: as his 2008 New Year's resolution, he decided to write a *thank-you note* a day for the rest of the year to everyone he knew.

Kralik's 2008 "gratitude project" had changed his

life completely. Instead of his feeling of discontent regarding his lack, and his envy of those who had what he did not have, he had learned to be *grateful* for his law firm, his practice, his friends, and his family, despite the many disasters and drawbacks he had previously experienced. Kralik's gratitude began to change every aspect of his life. His relationships with his family, his friends, and his staff improved significantly; his law firm avoided bankruptcy, and turned around completely.

Gratitude is something that you get more only by giving it away more. Expression of gratitude generates happiness that overcomes the unhappy feelings of lack.

Generosity

Be generous with your time, your labor, and whatever you may have. Show generosity to others around you.

Form the habit of giving without expecting any credit, recognition, or anything in return for your generous gesture. If you give with the intent of receiving, you become a "user" and not a real "giver."

Generosity does not necessarily have to do with giving or spending money. It is not solely based on your own economic status or how much money you have, but on your pure intentions of looking out for society's common good and giving from the bottom of your heart. Generosity should reflect your passion to help others who are in need, or who are less fortunate than yourself.

Mother Theresa once said that it is more blessed to give than to receive. According to **Buddha**, generosity is one of the Ten Perfections, which are human virtues cultivated as personal purification to live an unobstructed life for spiritual enlightenment.

Giving generosity is spiritual giving because God is giving. He gave man life itself (**Acts** 17:25), He constantly sustains man by His providential gifts (**Acts** 14:17), and, most significantly of all, He gave His beloved Son so that man may have eternal life (**John.** 3:16; **Romans** 6:23). If God is generous, so should you be!

> One gives freely, yet grows all the richer;
> another withholds what he should give,
> and only suffers want. Whoever brings
> blessing will be enriched, and one who
> waters will himself be watered.
> (**Proverbs** 11:24-25)

So, always be generous with your time, your care, your love, your understanding, and your forgiveness. Generosity will forever change your perceptions of life and living, especially your connectedness with others. Generosity is a necessity, not a luxury, in the miracle of life and living.

Sympathy and Empathy

Misfortunes and tragedies now and then happen along anyone's life journey. Their occurrence may also serve another life purpose: providing humans with an opportunity to offer their sympathy and empathy toward their fellow human beings. Sympathy and empathy are a fundamental people skill to show that they care about others, and not just about themselves.

Basically, we all have the inherent ability to know and understand what another person is feeling and experiencing, especially that person's deep pain and great suffering. Sympathy and empathy may bring out the best in humans in that they can express openly their care, concern, and comfort.

Sympathy and empathy, however, are not quite the same: the former shows *caring* about the pain and suffering of others, while the latter takes a further step in *feeling* the pain and suffering such that some actions have to be taken. Empathy, in particular, is often uplifting to the individual who is actually experiencing the pain and suffering, as well as infectious and inspiring to those around. Despite their apparent differences, both sympathy and empathy demonstrate comfort and support to those who are in need, and both lay the foundations for becoming a caring and compassionate person.

Compassion and Loving-Kindness

Empathy often leads to compassion and loving-kindness, which originates from the Hebrew, meaning the love and kindness of God freely given to man.

There is profound wisdom in expressing loving-kindness because it re-connects your soul or spirit to God.

> Who so is wise, and will observe these things, even they shall understand the loving-kindness of the LORD.
> (**Psalm** 107:43)

Loving-kindness is an act motivated by love, and freely expressed to your fellow human beings. To optimize this spiritual behavior, develop the mindset for compassion, which should become a habit or second nature to you.

To illustrate, when a person is not nice to you, your immediate response and reaction to that person may become habit-forming. Immediately, your mind tells you: "I won't let him or her step over me!" Over time, your response will become habitual and spontaneous— a natural way of expressing your individuality and your rights. In other words, it has become deeply etched in your soul. Always focus on developing a mindset for compassion, instead of asserting your individuality and your rights.

Showing compassion is not about "an eye for an eye" nor is it about your "rights" as an individual. Loving-kindness is an act of compassion that you *consciously* express to another individual simply because that individual has the same desire to be happy and to avoid suffering, just like yourself. Accordingly, your response is a *reflection* of your love for that individual, irrespective of the behavior of that individual toward you. However, that does not imply that you have to accept, approve, or even condone the inappropriate behavior of that individual.

Loving-kindness is just a positive response in your attempt to *change* the inappropriate behavior of that individual. The outcome of that attempt to change has nothing to do with your immediate response, because the attempt is out of your compassion and loving-kindness for that individual, irrespective of your success or failure in actually *changing* the behavior of that individual.

On the other hand, withholding loving-kindness may also be a mindset that you may have acquired through your culture or your repeated observation of similar responses by others toward similar behaviors in similar situations. Unfortunately, this toxic mindset may have seared your soul.

Fortunately, any bad behavior or inappropriate mindset can be changed or replaced by a positive one. Just *consciously* develop your own right mindset of compassion and loving-kindness to re-connect your soul or spirit to your Creator—just as **Dalai Lama**, the

Tibetan spiritual leader, once said: "Love and compassion are necessities, not luxuries. Without them, humanity cannot survive."

Toxic behaviors may come from toxic beliefs—such as one can do almost anything to be "street smart" as long as one is not breaking the law; one can justifiably step over someone while climbing one's own ladder of success.

Toxic emotions may come from one's wants and desires, such as envy and covetousness, anger and rage fuming over deprivation of one's desires, and among many others.

Toxic culture and environment may promote and endorse greed and lust for material things, and even addiction to speed.

But compassion and loving-kindness may also let you have better understanding of the toxic emotions of others around you. In their shoes, you may have more empathic feelings of *why* and *how* they behave or react in certain ways. Empathy is connectedness with other human beings, which is critical to maintaining good human relationships and sustaining the wellness of the mind and the spirit.

Dalai Lama shows how he instantly connects to people of different cultures, religions, and political perspectives. According to the Tibetan spiritual leader, on the very first meeting with any individual, he trains his soul to feel that the individual is simply another fellow human being with the same desire to be happy and to avoid suffering, just as he himself. With that mind-soul connection, he then becomes "connected" to everybody, without any exception, in the physical world.

With that same awareness, you may develop a positive mentality toward not only yourself but also others—which holds the key to improving human relationships and expressing compassion and loving-kindness to others around you.

C.S. Lewis, author and intellectualist, also shows how you, too, can "discipline" your mind filled with negative emotions. When you know that you are not going to behave friendly toward another person, you just *consciously* put on a much friendlier manner, such as a big smile, and behave as if you were a much nicer person than you actually are. In a few minutes, you may actually *feel* friendlier toward that person because you have just re-connected your mind to your soul, resulting in better behavior in your body.

<u>TAO wisdom</u>

According to **Lao Tzu**, "an eye for an eye" will only make you blind to the truth of oneness with all life—what goes around comes around.

> An eye for an eye
> makes us become what we hate.
> Knowing this, we do not
> rejoice in victory over our enemies,
> nor take delight in their downfall.
> Victory is but an illusion:
> getting even gains us nothing.
> (Lao Tzu, ***Tao Te Ching***, Chapter 31)

Lao Tzu even challenges us to ask ourselves these self-intuitive questions:

> Can we embrace both good fortunes and misfortunes in life?
> Can we breathe as easily as innocent babies?
> Can we see the world created as if without any judgment?

Can we accept both the desirable and the undesirable?
Can we express compassion to all without being boastful?
Can we watch the comings and goings of things without being perturbed?
(Lao Tzu, ***Tao Te Ching***, Chapter 10)

In a Nutshell

"Anything is everything" is all about subjective perceptions based on an individual's own perceived needs and wants. If the mental focus is too much on self, to the exclusion of all others, that individual may then become a frog in a well, with limited vision of anything and everything.

To jump out of the well, that individual requires both human wisdom and spiritual wisdom: the former is the knowing of one's true self; the latter is the looking beyond one's ego-self. Essentially, it is reaching out to others through connectedness based on the oneness with all life.

<u>TWO</u>

EVERYTHING IS NOTHING

Understanding is Everything

"Any fool can know. The point is to understand." **Albert Einstein**

Understanding is the ultimate truth of human existence. In the Christian tradition, truth begins with God, and not with self. However, in Eastern cultures, "understand self" is the *first* step in the pursuit of profound human wisdom.

Simply put, no matter what, humans are given a physical body, a mind, and a soul or spirit. The body lives in the material world, and is equipped with the five senses to live and survive in the physical environment. The mind, as the mediator between the body and the soul, is given the gift of free will, which is the freedom to process any input in the form of thoughts and sensations from both the body and the soul. That is to say, whenever we wish to do something, the soul intuitively provides the instinctive judgment, the mind then gives the analysis and the interpretation, and the body eventually executes the appropriate action or decision of the mind.

Therefore, the human mind plays a pivotal role in the understanding and the interpretation of some of these ultimate truths in human existence:

- The mind and the ego

- Attachments and illusions

- Control and power

- Detachment and letting go

- Impermanence and emptiness

The Mind and the Ego

"If a man thinks he is not conceited, he is very conceited indeed." **C.S. Lewis**

As soon as a baby begins his or her perceptions of the world through the five senses, that baby then begins to develop an identity, such as "this toy is *mine*" and "*I* want this and not that." There is nothing wrong with this initial identification. However, as time progresses, the identity of the baby then becomes the ego that continues to thrive, grow, and expand to the extent that it may become problematic, leading to the human flaw of attachments.

First, look at yourself in front of a mirror. What do you see? A *self* reflection in the mirror. Is it for real? Can you touch it? Not really; it is only a *reflection* of someone real—the real *you* in front of the mirror!

Now, do something slightly *different*. Place a baby—if there is one immediately available—in front of the mirror. See what happens next. The baby may crawl toward the baby in the mirror. Why? It is because the baby in front of the mirror thinks that the baby reflected in the mirror is *another* baby, and not him or her.

Likewise, the ego-self may look real, but it is *not* real. To think otherwise is only self-deception and self-illusion of the mind.

How the ego becomes anything and everything

Descartes, the great French philosopher, made his famous statement: "I think, therefore I am." So, you think and you then become what you *think* you are—the byproducts of all your thoughts and your own thinking.

Unfortunately, this famous statement by Descartes is only *partially* true: it is true that you identify yourself with your thoughts projected into your thinking mind; but it is *not* true that your identities thus created by your thoughts and your own thinking reflect your *true* self. The fact of the matter is that you are *not* your thoughts, and your thoughts are not *you*. To think otherwise is a human flaw, which is no more than just self-delusion or self-illusion. In other words, you are *not* what and who you *think* you really are, and that is *how* you may have created your own ego-self over the years.

A baby does not have an ego-self (at least, not yet), and thus sees the reflected image in the mirror as *another* baby; on the other hand, with your ego-self, you see the reflected image in the mirror as the *same* you, and not a *different* person other than you. Therefore, your ego-self is simply a reflection of you; what you see in the mirror is *not* real, just a reflection. But the problem is—you *think* it is the real *you*, and, wor*se*, you begin to *believe* it is.

As soon as the baby begins to learn how to perceive and interpret his or her own sensations through the five senses, those experiences will then get stored at the back of the mind as thoughts and memories—the raw materials with which the baby begins to create his or her own identity or ego-self. That is how a person's ego is formed.

Your mind, like a baby's mind, originally, was just like a blank sheet of paper. Your thinking begins with your five senses—*how* they perceive and interpret all your life experiences. All these physical and mental sensations then become your thoughts or memories stored at the back of your subconscious mind. Whenever you experience a similar sensation, your mind will automatically go back to your subconscious mind to look for more clues or relevant information, sending out different messages to your conscious mind, and instructing it to act or react accordingly. As an illustration, a baby, who previously experienced a pleasant sensation, will then begin to smile as soon as the subconscious mind sends to the conscious mind the very same message of that pleasant sensation previously experienced.

How it may become the human flaw

What is wrong with being the reflected person in the mirror?

For one thing, it is unreal. For another, if it is a positive image, you would expect to sustain that image; if it is a negative one, you would then strive to avoid being that image.

To illustrate, if you perceive yourself with a good body image; you may then try to do anything and everything to protect and sustain the positive image that has now become your ego-self. By the same token, if you look at yourself in the mirror and see an obese and negative image, you will have a deflated ego-self; you may then do anything and everything to bring about an improved body image in the future.

Well, there is nothing wrong with having an inflated or a deflated ego-self—whichever way you perceive, you may want to "exercise more" to protect or to improve that perceived body image of yours. There is nothing wrong with that. But any *attachment* to the ego-self may also create many other negative attachments, such as envy, regret, bitterness, frustration, and disappointment, which are only automatic and involuntary distorted thoughts that may prevent you from seeing your true self, and they thus ultimately become your human flaws.

To further illustrate the above point: say, you cooked a new dish for a potluck dinner; you liked its taste, and so did all your friends who complimented on your gourmet dish and asked for your recipe. These thoughts of compliments may have become registered in your subconscious mind. Consciously and subconsciously, you may then begin to actually "believe" that you *are*, indeed, a good cook. Slowly and imperceptibly, similar life experiences have begun to build up and reinforce your ego-self of being a gourmet cook.

As a result, you may begin to value only the past—reminiscing the taste of that gourmet dish and recalling all the compliments by your friends on that dish in the past; and now you also look forward to the future—projecting your mind into the future with expectations that your friends will continue to like and compliment that same gourmet dish. You may not even want to try creating another new dish for fear that it may not turn out to be as good as that gourmet dish in the past, or that it may not live up to the high standard of expectations projected by your mind into the future.

Isn't it true that nearly all of us are concerned with our past achievements, keeping the past *alive*—just look at all the awards, medals, and prizes we might have won over the past years—and projecting them into the future as desires and expectations of their continual recognition or fulfillment? The truth of the matter is that we all have identified ourselves not only with all our past achievements but also with our anticipated accomplishments in the future. We just want to continue feeling good about ourselves.

What is wrong with feeling good about ourselves, or wanting to continue with our past accomplishments and projecting them into the future as expectations? Well, this may lead to *over-doing*, which is doing more than what is necessary, and even to the extent of doing what might be wrong or even illegal.

<u>An illustration</u>

Lance Armstrong, the once-celebrated-but-now-disgraced cyclist, had won seven consecutive Tour de France titles and the Olympic bronze medal.

Armstrong's initial success inflated his ego that led to his craving for more future success, resulting in his "wrong doing"—using performance-enhancing drugs to win all his subsequent races that ultimately brought about his downfall, and he was stripped of all his previous winning titles.

Any obsession with a man-made identity may also lead to the comparison and contrast of self with others that only further distorts the perceptions of the human mind.

<u>An illustration</u>

There was an ancient Chinese fable of a stonecutter who worked so hard cutting stones that he often felt stressed and depressed.

One day, while standing behind a huge stone where he was cutting his stones, he looked up at the sky, and saw the beautiful sun. Then, he wished he were the sun that could give warmth and sunshine to everyone on earth. A fairy came to him and granted him his wish, so he became the sun.

For a while, he was happy and contented. Then, one day, a big cloud came over, blocked out everything from his view, and he could not even see what was below. He became distressed, and wished he were the cloud, instead of the sun. Again, the fairy came to his rescue, and granted him his wish. He became the cloud, and began drifting and floating happily and peacefully in the sky.

After a while, a strong wind came and scattered the cloud in different directions. Now, he wished he were the strong wind that could blow away anything and everything that stood in his way. Again, the fairy made his wish come true: he became the strong wind, blowing here and there. For a while, he was happy and contented.

Then, one day, he found that he could not blow away the big stone behind which he used to cut stones in the past. Worse, he was stuck there at the big stone, and going nowhere at all.

Now, finally, he realized that was where he belonged, and where he was supposed to be.

He made his one last wish to become the stonecutter that he used to be. The fairy granted him his last wish, and now he was contented to be the stonecutter again.

The moral of the fable: comparison and contrast between self and others is often a stumbling block to self-contentment, without which there is no self-discovery, which is the ultimate enlightenment. Self-acceptance is self-love—accepting yourself as who you are in spite of your shortcomings, without comparing and contrasting with others. Letting go of your ego-self is detaching yourself from your attachments that may ultimately become the sources of your miseries and sufferings in your life.

Remember, all human attachments come in the form of many different stressors in life, and are often the stumbling blocks in the human quest for true human wisdom because they create many illusions for the thinking mind.

Attachments and Illusions

"Attachment is the great fabricator of illusions; reality can be attained only by someone who is detached." **Simone Weil**

An attachment is no more than a safety blanket to overcome human fear—the fear of any change and the fear of the unknown from that change. To cope with that projected fear, you may just need many more attachments.

An attachment is basically your own emotional dependence on things and people that define your identity, around which you wrap your so called "happiness" and even your survival. Attachments are your holding on to anything and everything that you are unwilling to let go of, whether it is something positive or even negative.

We are living in a world with many problems that confront us in our everyday life and living, and many of these problems are not only unavoidable but also insurmountable. To overcome these daily challenges, many of us just turn to our own attachments as a means of distracting ourselves from facing our problems head on, or from adapting and changing ourselves in an ever-changing environment. All of our struggles in life, from anxiety to frustration, from anger to sadness, from grief to worry—they all stem from the same source: our attachment to *how* we want things to be, rather than relaxing into accepting and embracing whatever that might happen after we have put forth our own best effort.

Attachments often become the sources of human miseries and sufferings. Worse, they may come in many different forms that we are unaware of because of the illusions they have created in our minds.

Career attachments

Your career may span over several decades, involving many ups and downs, such as promotion and unemployment, changes of career and pursuits of higher qualifications, and among many others. They may all have become your problematic attachments.

Money and wealth attachments

Money plays a major role in life. You need money for almost anything and everything in life. In the past, people could enjoy some of the blessings of life without spending too much *real* money. Nowadays, to many people, enjoyment of life requires money—and lots of it—and you may be one of them. Attachment to money and the riches of the material world is often a result of an inflated ego-self. You may want to keep up with the Joneses—driving a more expensive car than the ones of your neighbors and friends.

Relationship attachments

Living has much to do with people, involving agreements and disagreements, often resulting in having mixed emotional feelings of joy and sorrow, contentment and regret, and among many others; they often become attachments to the ego-self as memories that you may refuse to let go of—not forgetting and not forgiving, for example, are some of the emotional hurdles that are often difficult for many to overcome.

Success and failure attachments

Success in life often becomes an attachment in the form of expectations that it will continue indefinitely, bringing more success. Failure, on the other hand, may generate regret, frustration, and disappointment. These emotional attachments are often difficult to let go of.

Adversity and prosperity attachments

In the course of human life, loss and bereavement are as inevitable as death. Loss can be physical, material, and even spiritual, such as loss of hope and purpose. You may want to attach to your good old days, and even refuse to let go of your current adversity. Both adversity and prosperity attachments also stem from the ego-self.

Time attachments

Time is a leveler of mankind: we all have only 24 hours a day, no more and no less, although the lifespan of each individual varies. Attachment to time is the reluctance to let go of time passing away, as well as the vain attempt to fully utilize and maximize every moment of time. This attachment often leads to the development of a compulsive mind and the action of over-doing.

The bottom line: sometimes we are so wrapped up in the outside world that we seldom have an opportunity to look inside of ourselves. Understanding who we really are may make us happy, instead of creating our own attachments in the material world we are living in. Imagine you are all alone in a room with *nothing*, except a pen and a piece of paper. Well, surprisingly, you may then become creative and even happy, with nothing there to worry about, and nothing there to distract your mind.

Identity crisis

According to **Tim Hiller**, a motivational speaker, a football coach, and a writer, "We usually don't realize the thing that is defining our identity until that thing is taken away."

Without attachments, we may all have an identity crisis; but the truth of the matter is that attachments only give us a false identity, and this may, ironically enough, lead to an identity crisis.

The spiritual wisdom is that **Jesus Christ** did not have an identity crisis: He clearly knew who He was; He never claimed to be someone else that He was not; He knew where He originated from, and also where He would be going. The problem with humans is that we do not know who we really are; through comparison and contrast, we strive to be someone else. Sadly, in the process, a *real* identity crisis ensues.

Attachment illusions

All human attachments are the raw materials with been which we both consciously and subconsciously create our own identities through a period of confusion and uncertainty that may eventually lead to not only the identity crisis but also the attachment illusions that distort our perceptions of the realities of life. Without human attachments, there will be no identity crisis, and no illusion of the mind.

For example, does the attachment to money bring happiness?

To many, it does, especially if they have been experiencing the lack of it! That explains why so many thousands of people line up for hours to get their lottery tickets, hoping against hope that their tickets would win them great fortunes, and hence bring them their happiness. But the reality is that many lottery winners claim that their happiness from the winning is only transient and is not lasting.

Bruce Lipton, author and cellular biologist, once said: "The function of the mind is to create coherence between our own beliefs and the reality that we experience. We generally perceive that we are running our lives with our own wishes and our own desires. But neuroscience reveals a startling fact: we only run our lives with our creative, conscious mind about 5 percent of the time; 95 percent of the time, our life is controlled by the beliefs and habits that are previously programmed in the subconscious mind."

It is your pre-programmed subconscious mind that tells you money can give you happiness. That can also explain why you may find yourself working in jobs that you do not even like due to your subconscious belief that money is anything and everything in your life.

The whole world out there that you see in front of you right now is nothing more than a projection of what you feel deep inside. Not only is it a projection of your deep feelings but also you internal energy. Yes, money is energy too, just like you, me, anything and everything else. Money is an expression of energy of your subconscious mind, building a complex system of money beliefs, such as "money makes the world go round" and "when I have enough money . . . then I'll be happy, and can do whatever I want to do."

But according to *Harvard Business Review*, money and happiness are not positively correlated, because money may make people *less* generous and *more* demanding and domineering. In addition, money may not bring out the best of an individual: the more money that individual has, the more focused on self that individual may become, and the less sensitive to the needs of people around, as well as the more likely to do the wrong things due to the feeling of right and entitlement.

The bottom line: any attachment to money only creates an illusion in the mind.

<u>An illustration</u>

Barbara Woolworth Hutton, also known as "the poor little rich girl", was one of the wealthiest women in the world during the Great Depression. She had experienced an unhappy childhood with the early loss of her mother at age five and the neglect of her father, and thus setting her the stage for a life of difficulty in forming relationships.

Married and divorced seven times, she acquired grand foreign titles, but was maliciously treated and exploited by several of her husbands. Publicly, she was much envied for her lavish lifestyle and her exuberant wealth; privately, she was very insecure and unhappy, leading to addiction and fornication.

She died of a heart attack at age 66. At her death, the formerly wealthy Hutton was on the verge of bankruptcy as a result of exploitation by others around her, as well as due to her own lavish and luxurious lifestyle.

She was the unhappy poor little rich girl! She was widely reported in the media, and her story was even made into a Hollywood movie: "The Poor Little Rich Girl."

The reality is that Barbara simply had too many attachments in her life: beauty, celebrity, fame, love, and above all, wealth—they had created too many illusions that they all ultimately brought about her unhappiness.

Remember, the more attachments you have, the

grater is your ego-self; unfortunately, an ego-self is not the *real* self, and so the so-called "happiness" is nothing more than just an illusion in the mind.

Control and Power

But why do all humans crave for attachments, always consciously and subconsciously wanting only more and more attachments to define who they are?

The answer is simple: humans want control and the power that often comes with control; they all want to control their own destinies through controlling others and circumstances.

Origin of control

Control is basic human instinct. Humans are inherently controlling. Out of fear and insecurity, our ancestors living as early as in the Stone Age strove to control their environment in order to survive, and thus developing their fight-or-flight instinct built in the human genes.

Since time immemorial, control has evolved, and most of us are controlling to a certain extent. We, as parents, control our children's destinies by striving to steer them clear of the wrong pathways we might have previously treaded ourselves. Our culture also tells us that we should be in control of anything and everything around us at all times, including our futures and destinies; controlling, to many of us, is synonymous with advancement and independence.

Irony of control

Stress in everyday life makes us want to control everyone and everything around us; ironically enough, in the process of controlling our stress, we may also inadvertently create for ourselves a vicious cycle of stress-generating-more-stress.

The anticipation of stress often puts us on an alert system, producing stress hormones. We then have to make some choices—choosing this or avoiding that so as to avoid the stress. But choosing in itself is stressful, especially picking the wrong choices, and thus leading to regret and disappointment. Even any expectation of the anticipated result may also intensify the stress, often making us do more than what is necessary in order to guarantee the expected result. Over-doing is stressful.

The irony is that *controlling* stress may only lead to getting more stress, and not less.

Ways of control

Control may come in many different forms in different phases in life, and we are all susceptible to exerting some forms of control. Given that control is basic human instinct, we *all* spontaneously want to control *how* people perceive us, especially if we have an inflated ego-self.

To illustrate, if you ask a child: "How old are you?", the child may answer: "Five years and four months", while extending his or her four fingers to highlight the "four months." The child wants to *control* your perception of him or her—that is. he or she is "four months" older than other five-year-old kids. If you ask a teenager the same question, that teenager may answer: "I am now fourteen"—implying that "I'm old enough to drive *soon*." But if you ask someone in the late twenties or early thirties the same question, that individual may answer quite *differently*: "I won't tell you; just *guess*!"—that individual is in fact trying to *control* your perception of his or her real age in relation to his or her appearance. If you ask an elderly person the same question, that person may be more willing to let you know his or her real age by saying: "I've just turned seventy!" That individual, too, is, in fact, *controlling* your perception: "See, I'm seventy, but I look much younger—probably like a fifty-year-old, don't I?"

In a way, we all want to *control* how people *think* of us. Do you like to wear loose-fitting clothing to hide your belly fat? Do you use heavy makeup to mask your facial lines? Do you dye your hair to make you look much younger? Control is about *changing* others' perceptions of your ego-self.

In addition to controlling how people perceive us, we may also want to control *how* people act and react toward us by using emotions, such as anger, fear, and guilt, and many other negative emotions. Furthermore, we may also want to control the circumstances we are living in, thereby controlling what is happening to and around us.

To a certain extent, we are all controlling in that we all have an ego-self with attachments that directly or indirectly control how people think and perceive, as well as how they act and react toward us.

Realities of control

Control is seldom welcome; rather, it is often received with aggression, alienation, and rejection. In addition, any controlling of self, of others, and of circumstances is, often than not, out of and beyond human control.

Divine inspiration

Whatever that is uncontrollable is divine inspiration with a lesson to learn.

<u>The parable and the real world</u>

In the famous Parable of the Prodigal Son (**Luke 15**), the younger son asked his father for his fair share of his estate. The father then gave him his fair share. With his fortune, the younger son traveled to a distant country, where he led a life of sin, and squandered all his fortune. His financial failure was followed by a natural disaster in the form of a famine. He learned the hard way that covetousness would not make him happy. Ultimately, he became penitent and returned to his father who welcomed him back.

The father was like God, letting a sinner go his own way, but would welcome him back with open arms if he becomes obedient and penitent, letting go of his covetousness.

In the real world, we, as parents, could *control* our son's destiny by not giving him his fortune, or setting up a trust fund so that he might not squander all his fortune. But there is no guarantee that he might not incur debts and still lead a dissipated and sinful life with no remorse. In other words, we can control only the money but we cannot control his destiny or how he squanders the fortune given or made available to him.

Dark side of control

What is wrong with controlling others, or even your own destiny? Control has its dark side: it expands your ego-self, and thus demanding only many more attachments; control is also the underlying cause of many human conflicts.

The bottom line: detach yourself from your ego-self as much as possible so as to let go of some, if not all, of your attachments in the material world in order to let go of your control of anything and everything.

Detachment and Letting Go

Humans are given a choice: continuing to control their destinies, or letting go of their control to let God control.

Detachment

Detachment is the beginning of letting go of anything and everything in life. But letting go is not easy, and is never appealing. It is because letting go means *change*, and any change is challenging, and therefore undesirable and unwelcome to many.

But detachment is the only way to go. Detachment begins with *awareness*—which is consciousness of thinking in the now. Becoming mindful of your body in the present moment is putting your mind where your body is. This awareness is deep relaxation for both your body and your mind—giving you the clarity of thinking to see and understand *how* and *why* you may have all your attachments in the first place. More importantly, your awareness may also enlighten your mind with simplicity in living by focusing more on the little things instead of on all the big things in your everyday life, and thus instrumental in initiating your letting go of anything and everything in life.

Wisdom of letting go

God has given each one of us a unique life and destiny that only *we* can complete it.

> Your eyes saw my unformed body; all
> the days ordained for me were written in
> your book before one of them came to
> be.

(**Psalm** 139: 16)

However, the completion of that life and destiny in our life journey is according to His way and time, and not according to ours. In other words, it is all about what He wants for us, and *not* about what we want for ourselves.

Get the spiritual wisdom of letting go of all your material attachments.

An illustration

Ann Russell Miller was a celebrated socialite from San Francisco, also known as **Sister Mary Joseph**. She, who had ten children and nineteen grandchildren, had grown up in luxury and privilege, and had been living a life of incredible wealth. Instead of shopping at Saks Fifth Avenue as she used to do for the past several decades, she suddenly decided to give up anything and everything in order to become a nun devoted to living in poverty for the rest of her life.

That unbelievable event happened more than two decades ago: one day, she held a celebrity party in which she announced her incredible decision, and her announcement was widely reported in the media across the United States.

Why did she make such an incredible decision to drastically change her lifestyle?

She said that she had a calling, a true vocation that was hard to understand for the general public, and even for the close members of her family.

Letting go of wealth is difficult because there is one thing that many of us fail to grasp and understand: money integrity.

The real value of money is its *integrity*. This is an important quality that can influence your value of money, in particular, all your financial decisions.

Integrity is to value what life has to offer, and not the things that can be purchased with money. Integrity is money wisdom. Remember, life has a great deal to offer, and some of the best things in life are free, such as your ability to think, to reason, to learn, and to live according to your destiny. Money is only a means to an end, but not an end in itself.

Maybe Ann Miller was suddenly awakened to the *real* meaning of her life without any of her material attachments, and subsequently to the spiritual wisdom of letting go in order to live the spiritual life of simplicity that was originally destined for her.

Trust and obedience

The burning question is: *How* do we know what God wants for *us*?

First and foremost, we must understand that the present mortal life on this earth is only secondary to the next immortal life yet to come. God has given each one of us a destiny—a unique role for each one of us to play on this earth. Accordingly, we are all wired with certain gifts and talents, desires and passions, characters and personalities, to live and function on this earth so that we may become what God has destined for us.

> And we know that in all things God works
> for the good of those who love him,
> who have been called according to his
> purpose.
> (**Romans** 8: 28)

God has also given us the free will to choose His perfect will, or to act according to what we want and desire for ourselves. Letting God means complete *trust* and *obedience*.

Trust in God means believing in the veracity of His Word.

> so is my word that goes out from my
> mouth:
> It will not return to me empty,
> but will accomplish what I desire
> and achieve the purpose for which I sent
> it.
> (**Isaiah** 53: 11)

Obedience to God means accepting and embracing any adversity and calamity in life so that we may learn lessons from them, thereby enhancing our spiritual wisdom to continue on our pathways to further trust and obedience.

> Teach us to number our days,
> that we may gain a heart of wisdom.
> (**Psalm** 90:12)

The miracle of letting God

God is in absolute control of anything and everything in the world that He has created.

> He says, "Be still, and know that I am
> God;
> I will be exalted among the nations,
> I will be exalted in the earth."
> (**Psalm** 46:10)

Throughout ages, miracles have happened around the world—a testament to the indisputable fact that God is always in control, despite humans' resistance to letting go of their futile endeavors to control their own destinies.

<u>An illustration</u>

Norbert Gennep, born in AD 1080, came from a wealthy and influential family in Germany, with ties to the imperial court. At that time in history, it was not uncommon for those seeking political advancement to also acquire ecclesiastical offices. So, Norbert had himself ordained a sub-deacon and became a canon, although he had no real piety or religious inclination; his ultimate motive was to indulge himself in worldly luxuries and pleasures.

Then, one day in AD 1112, while riding on horseback, he was struck by a fierce lightning, thrown from his horse, and remained unconscious for a while. On waking up, he was completely transformed, and asked: "Lord, what do you want me to do?" He heard God's voice, saying: "Turn away from evil, and do good." Obediently, he gave up everything he ever owned, became a priest, preached the Gospel, and lived the simple life of a wandering preacher in barefoot. He eventually became the Archbishop of Magdeburg in Germany, and was subsequently made a Saint by the Roman Catholic Church.

We do not have to be struck by lightning and thrown off the horseback before we would let go of our attachments to the material world, as well as our futile attempt to control our own destinies. God can work miracles in our lives if we are obedient, and if it is also His will.

Impermanence and Emptiness

Fact of impermanence

Impermanence is an inescapable fact of all human existence, clearly evidenced in the process of falling sick, growing old, and dying in all humans, as well as in the process of decaying of all things perishable and the passing away of anything liable to pass. There are no exceptions, and that is the indisputable fact of impermanence of anything and everything.

Perspectives of impermanence

According to **Buddha**, life is like a river. The water flowing in a river is like a progressive and a successive series of different but unified movements of water, all joining together to create the impression of one continuous flow of water. Likewise, human existence is moment to moment, with each moment leading to the next. It is an illusion that the person in this moment is the same person in the next moment; just as the river of yesterday is not quite the same as the river of today. To think otherwise is human illusion.

Even from a scientific point of view, Buddha's perspective is true. We know that cell divisions take place in each living being continuously: old cells in our bodies die and are continuously replaced by new ones. Technically speaking, all individuals are constantly subject to change, and the change is a continuous movement, just like the flowing water in a river.

Essence of change

The Creator has created for us a world of constant changes: everything is changing with every moment, remaining only with that very moment, and nothing remains permanent. It is through changes that we may transform ourselves into a better individual. Even in a difficult and challenging environment, we may learn from our mistakes and wrong choices in life, and so change ourselves. Change is transformation, which is educational and self-enlightening. Transformation is synonymous with impermanence, which is the essence of change.

Understanding that everything is impermanent is self-enlightening. Nothing is permanent: the good as well as the bad things that happen to us are impermanent; nothing lasts forever. We all are aware of this universal truth of impermanence. We all know that we cannot live to well beyond one hundred years, and yet we resist our aging process, continuously fixing our faces and bodies to make them look younger. We may have the face of a forty-year-old but the body and the mind of a seventy-year-old. We simply refuse to let go of the impermanence of all things; we desperately and self-delusively cling on to the "permanence" of all our attachments.

The illusion or self-delusion is that many of us wish the impermanent were the permanent. It is this wishful thinking that makes us unhappy. We were once healthy and now our health has declined, and we are unhappy. We were wronged by our enemies, and we still hold on to our old grudges, instead of forgiving and letting them go, and we are unhappy. Our past glories gave us the ego, which we refuse to let go of, and we become depressed and unhappy.

Life is about changes, and living is about letting go of what is impermanent that we naively believe and wish to be permanent.

Remember, nothing is permanent, and each and every moment remains only with that very moment. Therefore, live in the present, and live all your moments to their best and to the fullest as if everything is a miracle.

Permanent truths

Impermanence and change are the undeniable and permanent truths of all human existence. What is real is the existing moment, the present moment that is a product of the past, or a result of the previous causes and actions. Due to ignorance, an ordinary mind may conceive them all to be part of one continuous reality. But the fact that they are *not* is the permanent truth.

The various stages in the life of a man, the childhood, the adulthood, the old age are not the same at any given time. The child is not the same when he grows up and becomes a young man, nor when the young man turns into an old man. The seed is not the tree, though it produces the tree, and the fruit is also not the tree, though it is a product of the tree. This is the permanent truth of all life.

Emptiness and nothingness

Death empties anything and everything—that is, the ego and all its attachments to the material world. Emptiness is nothingness in which everything becomes nothing.

For all human efforts, death will come in the end for all and sundry. This is an indisputable fact. No matter how long a life you may want to live, you will, like everyone else, face dying one day. This is the way of all flesh because you have a built-in mechanism in your genes to ensure your mortality.

<u>Perspective of death</u>

According to **CNN** news, **Cathrin Ertmann**, a celebrated photographer from Denmark, chronicles the enigmatical journey of the deceased from death until burial. While keeping all her subjects' identities anonymous, she diligently records all the different stages of death, including autopsies and cremations, in quiet detail.

Before she started photographing death, Cathrin

Ertmann had never seen a dead body. Viewed through her lens while standing in a quiet morgue, it was, surprisingly, much less frightening and more of a quiet mystery for her to explore death and its implications.

"I was amazed about how peaceful and undramatic everything looked," she said. "I got the chance to look at death without it being my own relatives, without feelings involved, and it gave me a peace. The imagination of what death looks like is way worse than what I experienced. . . . . . I also saw a peace and beauty. Sometimes the scare is in the brief look at something. Like when you watch a horror movie, you only see a glimpse of the ghost, murderer or monster, and your imagination works all the fright up for you. I think I felt I need to see everything to make it 'normal' and undramatic. And I think it works the same way with our relation to death in general."

A new study of death gave Cathrin Ertmann a new perspective on life. "After working in the morgue, I was walking in the street and I got really over-whelmed by seeing all the people just walking, chatting and laughing," she said. "I wanted to yell: YOU ARE ALIVE, USE IT!"

Indeed, death is a leveler of all. We all have a life; so go out and live it as God has intended and planned for you.

> You will have to work hard and sweat a lot to produce the food you eat.
> You were made out of the ground. You will return to it when you die.
> You are dust, and you will return to dust.
> (**Genesis** 3:19)

The news on death by Catherin Ertmann is very illuminating: it sheds light on how we should all view death—or rather life and death, which are always interrelated. Remember, life always begets death, and what goes up must also come down. This is the natural cycle of anything and everything in this world. Many people live without ever thinking of death or deliberately ignoring its existence, while others live but always with death on their minds—especially those elderly. That death is inevitable is an indisputable fact, but one need not anticipate it as if it is imminent, even if one is advanced in years. Nobody knows when death may descend. Just live your life as if there is no tomorrow, live in the now, and live as if everything is a miracle.

Remember, whether or not you would like to let go of your attachments in the material world, you came from dust, and dust you shall return to.

> Remember your Creator
> before you return to the dust you came from.
> Remember him before your spirit goes back to God who gave it.
> (**Ecclesiastics** 12: 7)

The bottom line: remember your Creator, or where you came from; everything is nothing in the end. So, why hold on to, and why not let go of, anything and everything that eventually will become nothing? Just let go to let God, who is in absolute control; anything and everything must return to Him as nothingness. Indeed, the wisdom of *everything is nothing* is the wisdom of letting go to let God.

Death is emptiness, which brings an end to anything and everything in life. This emptiness, however, may have both positive and negative perspectives.

A glass-half-empty perspective of emptiness

Ernest Hemingway's famous novel *A Farewell to Arms* may show you a glass-half-empty perspective of emptiness:

> Once in camp I put a log on top of the fire and it was full of ants. As it commenced to burn, the ants swarmed out and went first toward the centre where the fire was; then turned back and ran toward the end. When there were enough on the end they fell off into the fire. Some got out, their bodies burnt and flattened, and went off not knowing where they were going. But most of them went toward the fire and then back toward the end and swarmed on the cool end and finally fell off into the fire. I remember thinking at the time that it was the end of the world and a splendid chance to be a messiah and lift the log off the fire and throw it out where the ants could get off onto the ground. But I did not do anything but throw a tin cup of water on the log, so that I would have the cup empty to put whiskey in before I added water to it. I think the cup of water on the burning log only steamed the ants.

The hero in the story was observing how the ants were swarming back and forth on a log on top of a fire in a futile attempt at survival—just like God watching over mankind's stubborn struggle to refuse letting go of the impermanent in the material world. Instead of acting as a messiah to help the ants, the hero emptied a tin cup of water so that he could have his whiskey.

The hero's attitude to death is also a reflection of the author's own perspective of man's ultimate fate: death happens no matter how hard one strives to avoid it, and anything and everything then becomes *nothing*.

Sadly and tragically, author Ernest Hemingway—essentially an atheist, although initially a Catholic—shot himself with a gun when he realized that anything and everything in his life was really *nothing*; with his perspective of nothingness, he had lost hope of human existence, including his own.

<u>A glass-half-full perspective of emptiness</u>

Francis of Assisi, the Italian Saint who chose a life of poverty in spite of his family's wealth, said on his deathbed: "Death will open the door of life." He died gracefully, while *singing*.

To Francis, emptiness is *everything*. Maybe for a believer, death is, indeed, a triumph, a meaningful exodus from this mundane world to the eternal world beyond. The emptiness is just a rite of passage to *everything*.

The wisdom is that without the Creator, you would have no life at all, only nothingness when death strikes in the end. Outside of the Creator, there is no reality. Everything was created for Him. Without the Creator, everything becomes nothing in the end. Without the Creator, Hemmingway viewed life as *everything is nothing*, despite all his fame and accomplishments, and he thus killed himself.

But, with the Creator, you may have *everything* because the nothingness then becomes everything in the life to come, and that explains why Francis of Assisi was singing on his deathbed.

In a Nutshell

You think, and you then become what you think; your thoughts are the raw materials with which you create your own ego-self.

But the ego-self is *not* your real self. Your ego-self only creates your own attachments in the material world to define who you wish you were.

Attachments are illusions of power to control what is uncontrollable, because anything and everything in this material world is impermanent.

Detachment may enlighten the human mind to let go of anything and everything, and to intuit the wisdom that nothingness may be *everything*.

THREE

NOTHING IS EVERYTHING

The Paradox

"I am the wisest man alive, for I know one thing, and that is that I know nothing." **Plato**

"The paradox of reality is that no image is as compelling as the one which exists only in the mind's eye." **Shana Alexande**

"The thinker without a paradox is like a lover without a feeling: a paltry mediocrity." **Soren Kierkegaard**

"Nothing is everything" is a paradox. In life, there are many paradoxes. The way of paradoxes is the way of attaining the ultimate truths of anything and everything. Knowing and understanding a paradox requires wisdom to see different human perspectives in anything and everything.

Paradoxes may be the way to wisdom, to the miracle of life, and ultimately to enlightenment.

<u>An illustration</u>

Christopher Paul Gardner, an American author,

entrepreneur, investor, and philanthropist, was very poor and homeless in the early 1980s. Sleeping on the floor of a public toilet, Gardner never dreamt that he would become a multi-millionaire one day. His inspiring life story was made into a hit Hollywood movie: "The Pursuit of Happyness."

Gardner was brought up with the belief that he could do or be anything that he wanted to do or be. At some point in his life, he was homeless; everything seemed nothing, just emptiness and nothingness, to him. But he was not hopeless. He continued to dream of wealth and success, and his dreams were not mirages. Because of his right doing and right thinking, he made his dreams come true.

Initially, Gardner made his living by selling medical equipment. He did not make enough money to make both ends meet, and his poverty made him homeless for a year.

Then, one day, Gardner met a stockbroker in a red Ferrari, who offered him internship because of his incredible drive and sustained enthusiasm. Thus he began his own successful investment career, and he subsequently even opened his own investment firm, Gardner Rich & Co.

More than two decades later, after the death of his wife, who challenged him to find his *true* happiness and fulfilment in the remainder of his life, Gardner made a complete career change. He was suddenly awakened to the notion that his fame, success, and wealth seemed like *nothing* to him then. His feeling of *nothingness* transformed him completely: he then became a philanthropist and a motivation speaker traveling around the world, focusing not on his own wealth, but on humanity and the needs of others to pursue their own happiness.

According to Gardner, life journey is always a process of lesson learning and forward moving:

"People often ask me would I trade anything from my past, and I quickly tell them *no*, because my past helped to make me into the person I am today." Yes, *nothingness* could be *everything* to him.

On any life journey, mental focus is essential: focusing not just on the big things in life but also on the small things as well; appreciating what you have, rather than dwelling on what is your nothingness.

What seems to be nothingness in the eyes of the world, when properly valued and put to use, can become anything and everything in the eyes of the beholder. Gardner turned his nothingness into great wealth. His ultimate enlightenment came when he looked at his own wealth in a different perspective—as no more than just *nothingness*—when he began to refocus his life goals on humanity and on inspiring others to become who they really are.

The bottom line: with wisdom you may know and understand the "nothing is everything" paradox that opens the door to self-enlightenment.

The Way

TAO, the profound wisdom of **Lao Tzu**, is the way toward knowing and understanding self and others, as well as things and circumstances around self. It may or may not lead to self-enlightenment, but at least it may help you *see* things as they really are, and not as they should be.

> Not knowing the Way,
> but pretending we know,
> we remain ignorant, and suffer.
>
> Knowing that we do not know,
> we pursue its wisdom:
> knowing its origin,

knowing its ending,
and knowing our true nature.
(Lao Tzu, **Tao Te Ching**, chapter 71)

TAO wisdom begins with emptiness, or more specifically, with an empty mindset.

The emptiness

Enlightenment has its origin from emptiness. Irrespective of whether or not attaining self-enlightenment, *emptiness* is the way to go toward attaining profound wisdom of living in this material world.

Emptiness is a way of human perception: looking at life experiences without adding anything to them, or without taking away anything from them. It is the thinking of the mind with no assumption and no presumption—that is, only an empty mindset.

As previously mentioned, emptiness can be either positive or negative (the glass half-full, or the glass half-empty). Positive emptiness can only occur when you allow yourself to surrender completely to any given circumstance or situation without any previous attachment.

According to **Lao Tzu**, develop an empty mindset, which is more than just "thinking out of the box": it is your *reverse* thinking to create your own empty box of thinking.

An empty mind with no craving and no
expectation helps us letting go.
Being in the world and not of the world,
we attain heavenly grace.
With heavenly grace, we become pure
and selfless.

And everything just settles into its own
perfect place.
(Lao Tzu, ***Tao Te Ching***, chapter 3)

An illustration

There was the story of a professor visiting a Zen master to find out more about Zen, which is an Eastern philosophy. In the beginning of the visit, the professor kept on talking, while the Zen master served him tea. At some point, the Zen master kept pouring tea into the teacup held by the professor even though it was brimming over. The moral of the story is that you must have an empty mind before you can accept new and unconventional ideas. Likewise, to intuit true human wisdom, you must have an empty mind capable of reverse thinking to find out the ultimate truths of anything and everything.

An empty mindset frees you from the many shackles of life that may have enslaved you and kept you in bondage without your knowing it. To be the master of your own life, you must have complete control over your own thinking mind, which must be empty without any pre-conditioned thoughts.

How do you gain control of your life in terms of your career, human relationships, time management, and daily stress, and among many others? First and foremost, you must empty your pre-programmed mind of any beliefs, blueprints, and roadmaps that tell you to do this or not to do that.

To illustrate, in your subconscious mind, you must set goals; to reach your goals, you must exert efforts; after accomplishing one goal, you need to set another higher goal, and yet another one higher than the previous ones; in addition, you must also have a role model to follow. But to take complete control of your life, you must empty your mind of all these pre-conditioned thoughts that are no more than your own attachments in the material world.

> When there is abundance,
> there is lacking.
> When there is craving,
> there is discontentment.
> Striving for power to control and
> influence every aspect of our lives
> is the source of our sufferings.
>
> Obsessed with getting and keeping,
> many of us never really live before we
> die.
>
> Following the Way,
> we must learn to let go of everything.
> (Lao Tzu, **Tao Te Ching**, chapter 75)

Life is always complex, and contemporary living is complicated with its many emotional and material clutters and attachments. To live well, you must learn to let go of anything and everything. The desire for simplicity may accelerate the process of letting go as life progresses. An empty mind with reverse thinking may help you let go of all your attachments in the complex and complicated material world you are living in.

But how can you attain an empty mindset?

Simplicity is the first step toward detachment, which is the key to unlocking the door to happiness. Live a simple lifestyle, deleting all the trimmings of life and living.

> Simplicity is clarity.
> It is a blessing to learn from those
> with humble simplicity.

Those with an empty mind
will learn to find the Way.

The Way reveals the secrets of the
universe:
the mysteries of the realm of creation;
the manifestations of all things created.
The essence of the Way is to show us
how to live in fullness and return to our
origin.
(Lao Tzu, **Tao Te Ching**, chapter 65)

Simplicity also shows you the true nature of all
things.

The Spirit is just like water flowing to all
things.
Its true nature is to give life
indiscriminately to all.
It flows to low places, where people
reject and despise.
It flows like a river, nurturing everything
and everyone on its way.
Its final stop is the ocean, which is its
very origin.

Living by the Spirit, we choose a simple
and humble lifestyle.
We meditate to enhance our spirituality.
We love our neighbors as ourselves.
We express compassion to all.
We speak with truth and sincerity.
We live in the present moment.
We take action only when necessary.

Without much ado or over-doing, we
trust the guidance of the Spirit.

In this manner, life flows like water, fulfilling itself and also everything naturally.
(Lao Tzu, ***Tao Te Ching***, chapter 8)

To further enhance an empty mindset, you need *mindfulness*, which is acute mental awareness of self and others, as well as of your own needs and not just your wants.

The mindfulness

Mindfulness is mental sharpness to know what is happening in the mind, and that brings about clarity of thinking, which is essential to attaining human wisdom. Mindfulness begins with the body. Becoming mindful of your body in the present moment is putting your mind where your body is.

watchful, like a man crossing a winter stream;
alert, like a man aware of danger;
courteous, like a visiting guest;
yielding, like ice about to melt;
simple, like a piece of uncarved wood;
hollow, like a cave;
opaque, like muddy water.
(Lao Tzu, ***Tao Te Ching***, chapter 15)

The now

According to **Lao Tzu**, only the present is real: the past was gone, and the future is uncertain and also unpredictable. When your mind stays in the now, you may not see your ego-self because it does not exist in the now, and only in your deceptive mind, which often focuses on the past, while projecting it into the future as an expectation.

> Living in the present moment,
> we see all things that we must do.
> Without complaint and resistance, we do them accordingly.
> Without seeking control and recognition,
> we simplify what we need to do, however complicated they may be.
> Trusting in the Creator, we always under-do and never over-do.
> (Lao Tzu, **Tao Te Ching**, chapter 30)

In the now, with clarity of thinking, you may see the ultimate truths of self and of others, as well as of anything and everything around you. Living in the now is your awakening to the realities of anything and everything in the world you are living in.

> Living in the present moment,
> we find natural contentment.
> We do not seek a faster lifestyle,
> or a better place to be.
> We need the essentials of life,
> not its extra trimmings.

> Living in the present moment,
> we focus on the experience of the moment.
> Thus, we enjoy every aspect of simple living,
> and find contentment in everyone and in everything.

> Living in contentment,
> we grow old and die,
> feeling contented.

(Lao Tzu, **Tao Te Ching**, chapter 80)

Therefore, we focus on the present
moment,
doing what needs to be done,
without straining and stressing.

To end our sufferings,
we focus on the present moment,
instead of our expected result.
So, we follow the natural laws of things.
(Lao Tzu, **Tao Te Ching**, chapter 63)

Remember, human sufferings are the result of not
focusing on the present; focusing on the now may let
you see your own connection with the Creator.

The Creator is like an ocean.
It fills everything and everywhere.
It is the origin of life.
It never abandons its creations.
It accomplishes everything, but needs no
recognition.
It nourishes and cherishes all,
yet gives everyone the freedom to
choose.
It has no need for glory,
so it retreats to the background
and becomes inconspicuous.
Yet we all return to it.
And that is why it is great.
Its greatness needs no recognition.

Likewise, our greatness comes
not from our power or control,
but from our own true nature,
which is living as one with the Creator.

(Lao Tzu, **Tao Te Ching**, chapter 34)

Trusting the Creator, we concentrate on
the Creator.
Relying on ourselves, we focus on our
ego.

Our greatest suffering comes from
not knowing who we are, or to whom we
belong.
Our greatest unhappiness comes from
wanting more than what the Creator
provides.
Our greatest satisfaction of contentment
is the lasting satisfaction.
(Lao Tzu, **Tao Te Ching**, chapter 46)

The spontaneity

The truth of the matter is that everything in life
must follow a natural cycle, whether we like it or not,
and that we must be patient because nothing is within
our control, especially our destinies.

That which shrinks
must first expand.
That which fails,
must first be strong.
That which is cast down
must first be raised.

Before receiving, there must be giving.
This is called perception of the nature of
all things.
Soft and weak overcome what are hard
and strong.
(Lao Tzu, **Tao Te Ching**, chapter 36)

Spontaneity is the essence of the natural cycle. What goes up must eventually come down; life begets death; day is followed by night, just like the four seasons. Anything and everything follows the natural cycle.

> Allowing things to come and go,
> following their natural laws,
> we gain everything.
> Straining and striving,
> we lose everything.
> (Lao Tzu, **Tao Te Ching**, chapter 48)

Intuition of spontaneity is the knowing and the understanding of the *impermanence* of all things: nothing lasts no matter how humans strive to keep the impermanent permanent; anything and everything remains only with that very present moment, and ultimately all become *nothingness*.

> Strong winds come and go.
> So do torrential rains.
> Even heaven and earth cannot make
> them last forever.
> (Lao Tzu, **Tao Te Ching**, chapter 23)

The judgment and the separation

According to **Lao Tzu**, one should not judge others, nor should one separate oneself from others.

> The Creator never seems to do anything,
> yet all things are done accordingly.

> We stay in the very center of the
> Creator,

and refrain from controlling our own destinies.
Everything will evolve and fall into its natural place,
according to the natural laws of the Creator.

When there is no desire to be someone that we are not,
separated from our true nature designed by the Creator,
all things are in perfect balance and harmony.
(Lao Tzu, ***Tao Te Ching***, chapter 37)

Being non-judgmental holds the key to attaining balance and harmony in a world that is full of chaos and disharmony.

> Stop striving to be righteous and wise to attain salvation, which comes not from our efforts, not from something we must earn.
>
> Stop abiding by rules and regulations to secure fairness and justice.
> Compassion and loving-kindness come naturally to us.
> Stop accumulating riches by being smart.
> Heavenly assets are freely available to all.
>
> All of the above are merely superficial suggestions.
> The ultimate truths have to be self-intuited:

Be simple, be selfless, and be non-judgmental.
Enlightenment may arrive effortlessly.
(Lao Tzu, **Tao Te Ching**, chapter 19)

The choosing and the picking

Following the natural cycle of all things, you need not pick and choose. Picking and choosing is only sickness of your mind: the futility in striving to control what is essentially uncontrollable.

People naturally avoid loss and seek gain.
But with all things along the Way,
there is no need to pick and choose.
There is no gain without loss.
There is no abundance without lack.
We do not know how and when
one gives way to the other.

So, we just remain in the center of things,
trusting the Creator, instead of ourselves.
This is the essence of the Way.
(Lao Tzu, **Tao Te Ching**, chapter42)

Picking and choosing is synonymous with control of self, of others, and of anything and everything around, which is against the laws of nature.

Controlling external events is futility.
Control is but an illusion.
Whenever we try to control,
we separate ourselves from our true nature.
Man proposes; the Creator disposes.

Life is sacred: it flows exactly as it
should.
Trusting in the Creator, we return to our
breathing, natural and spontaneous,
without any conscious control.

In the same manner:
sometimes we have more,
sometimes we have less;
sometimes we exert ourselves,
sometimes we pull back;
sometimes we succeed,
sometimes we fail.

Trusting in the Creator, we see the
comings and goings of all things,
but without straining and striving to
control them.
(Lao Tzu, **Tao Te Ching**, chapter 29)

TAO wisdom is to embrace *all*, instead of choosing and picking this and that.

Good fortune and misfortune are all in
one.
Seeking one and rejecting the other,
we become completely confused.
Striving for goodness and righteousness,
we become evil and wicked.
(Lao Tzu, **Tao Te Ching**, chapter 58)

No picking and no choosing is the wisdom in seeing the dualism of anything and everything, such as "life and death" and "success and failure"—they all go hand in hand, and one ultimately becomes the other.

Accepting what is, we find perfection in

the Creator,
as well as in anything and everything
created by Him.

What seemingly distorted is in fact
truthful.
What seemingly lacking is in fact
abundant.
What seemingly exhausted is in fact
refreshing.

Possessing little, we become content.
Having too much, we lose the Creator.
Having no ego, we become humbled, and
our actions are enlightened.
Having no desire for perfection, our
actions are welcome by all.
Having no expectation of result, our
actions are selfless and non-judgmental.
Having no goal, our actions are under-
doing and never over-doing.

Accepting what is, and finding it to be
perfect is not easy.
But that is the Way to the Creator.
(Lao Tzu, **Tao Te Ching**, chapter 22)

TAO wisdom, however, does not imply that there is
no free will, or freedom of choice.

Fame or self, which is dearer?
Self or wealth, which is greater?
Gain or loss, which is more painful?

Accumulating or letting go, which causes
more sufferings?

Looking for status and security, we find
only sufferings.
Knowing our true nature, we find joy and
peace.
With nothing lacking, the whole world
belongs to us.
(Lao Tzu, **Tao Te Ching**, chapter 44)

Embracing anything and everything is beneficial because it holds the key to enlightenment, which is the understanding of the impermanence and the nothingness of anything and everything in the world we are living in.

The Way to the Creator has no blueprint.
With faith and humility, we seek neither
pride nor blame.
Our actions then become righteous and
impeccable.
Our lives are illumined with the Creator's
light.

Everything that happens to us is beneficial
Everything that we experience is
instructional.
Everyone that we meet, good or bad,
becomes our teacher or student.

We learn from both the good and the
bad.
So, stop picking and choosing.
Everything is a manifestation of the
mysteries of creation.
(Lao Tzu, **Tao Te Ching**, chapter 27)

The expectation and the doing

TAO wisdom emphasizes "wu-wei" (無為): "wu" (無) means "no" and "wei" (為) means "doing." Due to the literal translation of the original text, "wu-wei" is sometimes misinterpreted as "non-doing," and therefore even regarded as a "passive" way of looking at life by **Lao Tzu**. "No over-doing" is a more appropriate translation of "wu-wei."

Contrary to conventional wisdom, which focuses much on effort, TAO wisdom emphasizes "effortless" effort.

> The softest thing in the world
> overcomes what seems to be the
> hardest.
>
> That which has no form
> penetrates what seems to be
> impenetrable.
>
> That is why we exert effortless effort.
> We act without over-doing.
> We teach without arguing.
> This is the Way to true wisdom.
> This is not a popular way
> because people prefer over-doing.
> (Lao Tzu, **Tao Te Ching**, chapter 43)

With "effortless" effort, there is no over-doing; trust and obedience then come naturally, and everything is done.

> We act without over-action.
> We manage without interference.
> We enjoy without attachment.
> Effrontery is just
> an opportunity for loving-kindness.
> Great accomplishments are only

a combination of small steps.
Difficult tasks are no more than
a series of easy steps.
(Lao Tzu, ***Tao Te Ching***, chapter 63)

The humility and the ego

If TAO wisdom could be summarized in one word, it is the word "humility."

Humility is the enemy of the ego, while pride is its best friend. With humility, we see who we really are, and not who we think or wish we were. With humility, we become aligned with the Creator, who provides us with the wisdom in living in this material world. With humility, we do what is necessary, but without any over-doing. With humility, we do not pick and choose because we have no expectation of any outcome. With humility, we trust the Creator and believe in the spontaneity of anything and everything created by Him. With humility, we live in the present, in perfect harmony with self and with others around us. With humility, we are in the world, but not of the world.

Humility is power.
Power comes from the lowly.
According to the Way:
the lowly will be elevated;
the last will be the first.

The Creator is above,
and we are below.
The Creator is in front,
and we are behind.
Because this is the nature of things,
humility is only natural to us.
Yet many are desirous of the top
fearful of lagging behind.

Humility is the Way.
(Lao Tzu, ***Tao Te Ching***, chapter 66)

The bottom line: TAO is the way to anything and everything, and the Way is TAO wisdom.

The Way is easy,
yet people prefer distracting detours.
Beware when things are out of balance.
Remain centered within the Creator.

Distractions are many,
in the form of riches and luxuries.
They allure us from the Way.
Accumulations are like extortions of the poor.
They bring only disasters and sufferings.
Do not deviate from the Way.
(Lao Tzu, ***Tao Te Ching***, chapter 53)

According to **Lao Tzu**, this is how the human mind may have become distorted and dysfunctional:

- In the beginning, man did not know things existed, and so he had perfect knowledge.

- Later, he found out things existed, but made no distinctions between them.

- Then, he began to make some distinctions, but expressed no judgment about right and wrong.

- Now, he makes judgments of right and wrong, and that leads to his own preferences of likes and dislikes, which then create his desires and expectations—the sources of his sufferings. In short, the human mind is like an unbridled horse: it makes judgments, making what does not exist, exist, and what does exist, does not exist. In the process, illusions and self-deceptions are created, and they become the attachments or substances of the ego-self.

Accordingly, change the way you think through your mind to change the way you see the world, and your life will be totally different. Remember, the TAO mind is *not* the human mind. The human mind is concerned with material things and worldly life, forever making false distinctions and discriminations based on human desires to seek pleasures and to avoid pains. The TAO mind is a perfect mirror that reflects anything and everything perfectly, but it does not hold on to anything and everything at all, because what it sees in the mirror is just a reflection, an image of something intangible, unreachable, and therefore unreal. Use your mind like a mirror to reflect what you see, but without retaining it, and therefore you learn to let go of anything and everything that you see in the mirror, because it is unreal. That is the true wisdom in the art of living well.

A TAO mind, however, does not stop you from living a proactive life in this material world, but all your actions and activities should fit into the natural patterns of the universe, with complete detachment of your attachments to the ego-self.

Remember, life is not a mirror of anything and everything in your mind's eye.

Bottom line: TAO wisdom is the way to the miracle of life and living, but this profound human wisdom is not easy to self-intuit without the help and guidance of spiritual wisdom.

The Miracle

"The fear of the LORD is the beginning of knowledge; fools despise wisdom and instruction." **Proverbs** 1: 7

"Do all things without grumbling or questioning, that you may be blameless and innocent, children of God without blemish in the midst of a crooked and twisted generation, among whom you shine as lights in the world," **Philippians** 2: 13-15

"When the Spirit of truth comes, he will guide you into all the truth, for he will not speak on his own authority, but whatever he hears he will speak, and he will declare to you the things that are to come." **John** 16:13

Life is a miracle. Miracles happen everyday, but you just have to *open* your heart, mind and soul to *see* these miraculous encounters, that is. looking the *right* way.

Looking the right way, you will see: you have a unique destiny with a divine purpose designed only for you; you have many imperfections, just like everyone else, but they are your *connectedness* to all through love and compassion, as well as forgiveness; you are going to face many changes and challenges ahead of you that are meant only to transform you into a better being.

To ensure that you are always looking at the right way, you need faith, which is *belief*.

According to **St. Augustine**, the Bishop of Hippo (354-430 A.D.), in life there are certain things we do not believe unless we understand them, and there are other things that we do not understand unless we believe them. To St. Augustine, faith is not opposed to understanding, nor is it independent of understanding. His famous "faith seeking understanding" is an act of believing *first*, without which unbelief closes the door to any *further* understanding. "Belief to overcome unbelief" is another important paradox of life.

St. Anselm of Canterbury, a well-known Christian philosopher and theologian of the eleventh century, also echoed St. Augustine's statement in his famous motto: "I do not seek to understand in order that I may believe, but I believe in order to understand."

> By faith we understand that the universe was formed at God's command, so that what is seen was not made out of what was visible.
> (**Hebrews** 11: 3)

Accordingly, to begin your own spiritual journey of seeking God's wisdom, you must, first and foremost, have faith seeking knowledge to understand God with belief to close the door of unbelief.

Believe that God brought you here for a purpose that you may not know. He will keep you in His love as long as you trust Him. To demonstrate that trust, you have to be obedient, which means you have to let go of all your attachments that are no more than just distractions from your fear of the unknown ahead of you. He will make any trial in your life a blessing, teaching you a lesson He intends you to learn from it. He is giving you His grace to be bestowed on you. In His good time, He will deliver you—how and when you may not know, and this is the trust, without which there is no letting go.

Remember, an inflated ego does not solve your life problems; it only increases them with many more attachments. Letting go of your ego is the way to go. Attachments are no more than your emotional dependence on things, people, and thoughts that make your reluctant and resistant to letting go. But only letting go can create the "emptiness" to be filled by God's wisdom to help you let go to let God.

Do not waste your spiritual energy by striving to seek answers to many of those unanswered questions about unfairness, inequality, injustice, or many of the inexplicable things that happened in your life. Just accept and embrace the miracle of life, and God will take care of anything and everything for you. Just leave it to Him, and nothing slips through His vast net of love and mercy.

> Do not fret because of those who are evil
> or be envious of those who do wrong;
> for like the grass they will soon wither,
> like green plants they will soon die away.
> Trust in the LORD and do good;
> dwell in the land and enjoy safe pasture.
> Take delight in the LORD,
> and he will give you the desires of your
> heart.
> (**Psalm** 37: 1-4)

The Enlightenment

"Knowing others is wisdom, knowing yourself is enlightenment." **Lao Tzu**

"Enlightenment, joy, and peace can never be given to you by another. The well is inside you." **Thich Nhat Hanh**

"Enlightenment is not a change into

something better or more, but a simple recognition of who we truly already are."
Anonymous

Enlightenment is an endless process of *knowing* and *understanding* anything and everything that is simply there and is available to all since the beginning of time. It is like knowing that at sunrise you will see sunlight as long as you open your eyes; its presence is *permanent*—but you just have to *open* your eyes to see its presence, and even the blind can just *feel* the presence of the sunlight.

Li Ching-Yuan, a Chinese herbalist, martial artist, and tactical advisor, known for his extreme longevity of well over 200 years—which far exceeded the longest confirmed lifespan of 122 years of a French woman—gave his profound wisdom on enlightenment.

> Before I had studied Zen for thirty years,
> I saw mountains as mountains,
> and waters as waters.
> When I arrived with a more intimate knowledge,
> I saw that mountains are not mountains,
> and waters are not waters.
> But now that I have got its very substance,
> I am at rest.
> For it is just that I see mountains once again as mountains, and waters once again as waters.
> **(Li Ching-Yuan)**

Enlightenment is effortless and spontaneous. So, if you strive to know and understand anything and everything, the enlightenment may never come. But that does not matter because you may *already* have the wisdom to *see* that "mountains are *not* mountains, and waters are *not* waters." The truth of the matter is that your mental capability to see "mountains once again as mountains, and waters once again as waters"—which is the *enlightenment* itself—may or may not come to you now or even for the rest of your life. Enlightenment may still be important to you, but not *that* important. After all, many of us may all pass through life with some wisdom but without really attaining our self-enlightenment. Having said that, it is important that at least you see "mountains are *not* mountains, and waters are *not* waters"—which is already profound human wisdom.

Yes, illusion and delusion may go on indefinitely, but enlightenment may take only a moment. It is the very moment of consciousness without being self-conscious.

The realization that nothing is in fact everything gives you freedom and liberation from all your previous attachments. Letting go to let God is self-enlightenment. Returning to dust is actually the only pathway to *everything*; physical death is just a way station on the road to eternity, and that nothingness ultimately becomes *everything* in the life to come.

In a Nutshell

Enlightenment is wisdom that understands the paradoxes of life, such as: what goes up must also come down; abundance is emptiness; everything is nothing; nothingness is everything.

THE END

APPENDIX A

TAO TE CHING

Tao Te Ching (道德經) is an ancient Chinese classic on human wisdom, written by **Lao Tzu**, the Chinese sage, who was born more than 2,600 years ago. This unique piece of literature is one of the most translated books in human history and world literature. The book is a beautiful collection of Chinese wisdom poetry, in which the author expresses his wisdom in living life in all of its beauty and joy, as well as in all of its pain and sorrow. The language is simple and poetic, but controversial and paradoxical.

TAO (道), also known as The Way or TAO wisdom, originated from **Tao Te Ching**.

> My words are easy to understand
> and easy to perform,
> Yet no man under heaven
> knows them or practices them.
> (Lao Tzu,*Tao Te Ching*, Chapter 70)

There are altogether 81 short chapters, expressed in only 5,000 words. It must be pointed out that there was no punctuation mark in the original text. Given that each word in the Chinese language may have multiple meanings, the original text without any punctuation is open to many different interpretations —just like the story of the three blind men touching different parts of the same elephant, while describing what an elephant may look like.

A plausible explanation for the many different interpretations was that Lao Tzu was reluctant to express his wisdom in words. As a matter of fact, according to the legend, at that time he was at the point of leaving China for Tibet, when he was stopped at the city gate and was told by the guard that he had to put down his wisdom in words before he could leave the country. Deliberately and defiantly, he put down his wisdom concisely and precisely in only 5,000 words with no punctuation mark at all to show his defiance and reluctance.

TAO wisdom is profound human wisdom that requires self-intuition to have greater understanding of the Creator, who is in control of anything and everything created by Him; this further understanding may be instrumental in enhancing human wisdom. For this reason, paradoxically, TAO was later on evolved into a religion (known as Taoism) in China. However, it must be pointed out that TAO was never intended to be a religion or some religious belief by Lao Tzu; it was meant to show only what *true* human wisdom really is.

APPENDIX B

MINDFULNESS

"Wherever you go, there you are." **Jon Kabat-Zinn**

Consciousness

Mindfulness is purposeful consciousness of the present moment. Practicing mindfulness is your only pathway to your appreciating the present moment. Anything you experience after coming into presence through mindfulness may become richer and more meaningful to you. This is how and why mindfulness can give you better health and greater happiness.

In mindfulness, you recognize your thoughts as they occur, but you pay non-judgmental attention to them; in other words, they neither distract nor disturb you, and you just *observe* them, like watching a movie about yourself unfolding before your very eyes.

If you are conscious of what your body and your mind are experiencing in the present moment, you will soon learn how to become mindful of others, which is the beginning of compassion and loving-kindness—a quality that enriches life, making you happier, and maybe even wiser. If you are mindful of others, you will also become mindful of anything and everything in life, such as your breathing and your eating.

Breathing comes so natural that many of us are not even mindful of how we breathe. As a result, many of us do not breathe correctly, and we get less oxygen to our lungs, cells, and even to our brains. Likewise, eating becomes second nature to us that many of us are no longer mindful of the eating process: we simply shuffle and stuff food into our mouths, mindless of chewing and digesting the food we are eating. Indeed, in our daily routines, there are so many things that we are mindless about, because we have taken them for granted. Mindfulness is re-directing our attention to what we are doing at the present moment to re-establish our *consciousness*, which is the vital link between the body and the mind.

Practice the following to enhance your body-and-mind connection by putting your mind where your body is:

- Sit comfortably. Place the back of one hand in the palm of the other, allowing your thumb tips to touch lightly. Rest your hands on your body in line with your lower abdomen.

- Breathe consciously for a minute or two. Be aware of your breaths.

- Gently close your eyes. Focus your attention on the flow of your bodily sensations within your consciousness, such as the beating of your heart, the tingling and twitching of your muscles, as well as your sense experiences, such as the sounds, smells, and even tastes surrounding you.

- Meanwhile, thoughts may arise. Release them without any effort or struggle: just let them drift away. If need be, direct your attention back to your breathing, and again pay attention to the consciousness of all your physical sensations and experiences.

- Continue this process for as long as you like. You will feel the interconnection between your body and mind; it is the consciousness of your body that connects your body and mind in a unique way. Essentially, you are putting your mind where your body is in the present moment.

Mindfulness Walking

Walking is one of the best exercises to practice mindfulness. Be mindful of your walking: the walk must be brisk with full consciousness and deep concentration of the mind. Very often, we are so caught up with our destination that we put our feet into automatic pilot, while our minds drift from one thought to another. To stop our rambling thoughts, we must train our minds to concentrate through mindfulness while we are walking briskly.

Mindfulness walking requires you to pay full attention to what you are doing, to notice the movement of your limbs, the shifting of your body weight as you move your right foot and left foot. Mindfulness walking gives you an opportunity to quiet your mind, to practice subliminal messages, to enhance your mental concentration, and ultimately to empower your thinking mind.

Here is an example of how you can walk with mindfulness:

You can choose the first two verses from the famous **Psalm** 23: "**The Lord is my Shepherd. I shall not want.**" Repeat each syllable in your mind with each foot as you walk step by step, one step at a time. Always begin with your right foot, then followed by your left foot; continue your steps following each syllable with the corresponding right or left foot:

"The Lord is my She-pherd. I shall not want"
R   L   R L   R   L   R L   R   L

You always begin the first word with the right foot. So, if you have to begin the first word with the left foot instead, then you know you have messed up somewhere; in other words, you mind must have wandered off. When that happens, start all over again with your right foot first, followed by your left foot. You may be very surprised that even within a 10 to 20 minute walk you might have messed up the sequence and coordination several times, because your mind did not concentrate enough.

You can choose any other phrase or subliminal message to practice your mindfulness walking.

APPENDIX: C

MEDITATION

"The thing about meditation is that: You become more and more you." **David Lynch**

"Meditation brings wisdom: lack of meditation leads to ignorance. Know well what leads your forward and what holds you back, and choose the path that leads to wisdom." (**Buddha**)

Meditation is thinking about one thing at a time. Simple as it may seem, this requires practice and discipline. According to **St. Theresa of Avila**, the mind is like an unbridled horse wandering where it will, and your role is to train the horse, and gently and lovingly bring it back to the right course.

Meditation is training your mental attention to sharpen your *awareness* or *consciousness* of what is going on in your mind. Once you see clearly what is going on in the present moment, you can then choose to ignore or to act upon what you are seeing through your mind.

Meditation Basics

To meditate, you must get into the right frame of mind; that is, you must learn some meditation basics in order to know *how* to meditate effectively:

- You must be in a quiet environment conducive to meditation.

- Your body must be comfortable and still, and very relaxed.

- Your breathing must be right: inhale and exhale softly and slowly, preferably in a rhythm.

- Your mind must be focused, staying in the present moment, as much as possible.

- You must not expect anything to *happen* during your meditation session. You must practice with consistency and persistence.

How to Meditate

Find a quiet place where you can remain undisturbed for at least 20 to 30 minutes. To set the environment for meditation, you may want to have some scent from flowers or incense, or even some soothing music (meditation MP3) to enhance your senses. Of course, you can meditate without them; it is just an option, not a requirement.

Find time to practice meditation. Regularity holds the key to success in meditation. Do not meditate only when you feel like it. Find some quiet time for yourself every day. The ideal time to meditate is before retiring to bed; in that way, your mind can review what has happened during the day—what you have said and done—and then let go of everything. After all, meditation is about letting go of all the past and the future thoughts.

Correct posture is important. First of all, your

body must be erect: this induces correct breathing, which can bring all your internal energies into a state of harmony. Therefore, do not lean back on anything. If you find that your neck is too week or your spine cannot support your body, then rest your back on a hard surface initially; but the ultimate goal is to sit erect without your back touching anything.

You can sit cross-legged on the floor. Alternatively, you can sit comfortably on a chair (not a sofa), with your thighs at right angles to your spine, your hands on your thighs, your feet resting firmly on the floor, and your shoulders relaxed. In short, just sit "tall" and erect.

Always begin meditation with your breathing. Your breathing is an indicator of your stress level: if you are unduly stressed, your breathing becomes thick and gasping. Breathing right is your conscious control of stress. When you feel stressed, consciously change your breathing pace to undo the stress.

Gently close your eyes, or you can fix your eyes on an object.

As you begin your meditation, you will find that your first thought does not come to your mind right away. When it finally comes, do not dismiss it. Instead, *consciously* focus on your breathing. That thought will then slowly disappear. After a while, another thought or the same thought may come up to your mind. Again, do not consciously dismiss it; *refocus* on your breathing. With more practice, you will find that within a 10-minute time frame, fewer and fewer thoughts will crop up in your mind because your mind has stayed in the present moment for a longer period. The fewer thoughts you have, the more relaxed you may become. Then, one day, you may suddenly find that you have stepped into a totally different world with total tranquility and clarity of thinking—even though it may last but a very brief moment. That sensation is nondescript. Once you have attained that inexplicable and transformative state of mind, you will want to continue practicing meditation every day.

But do not expect that transcendental state of mind will come any time soon; the more you expect it to happen, the longer it will take you to attain that state of mind. Just consistently and patiently practice your meditation every day.

Meditation is life-changing. Meditation may change *how* you look at yourself and the days ahead of you.

APPENDIX D

WORDS OF WISDOM

"We are what we repeatedly do. Excellence, then, is not an act, but a habit." (**Aristotle**)

"The wise person questions himself, the fool others." (**Henri Arnold**)

"God asks no man whether he will accept life. That is not the choice. You must take it. The choice is *how*." (**Henry Ward Beecher)**

"When one door closes, another opens; but we often look so long and so regretfully upon the closed door that we do not see the one which has opened for us." (**Alexander Graham Bell**)

"We only live once, but once is enough if we do it right." (**Gary Ryan Blair**)

"Your work is to discover your work and then, with all your heart, to give yourself to it." (**Buddha**)

"What you are is what you have been. What you'll be is what you do now." (**Buddha**)

"Life is the art of drawing sufficient conclusions from insufficient premises." (**Samuel Butler**)

"Blessed are the hearts that can bend; they shall never be broken." (**Albert Camus**)

"All great changes are preceded by chaos." (**Deepak Chopra**)

"Courage is the first of human qualities because it is the quality which guarantees all the others." (**Winston Churchill**)

"Diseases of the soul are more dangerous and more numerous than those of the body." (**Cicero**)

"To know something is to know it; not to know something is not to know it. That is knowledge." (**Confucius**)

"It is not truth that makes man great.
But man that makes truth great." (**Confucius**)

"Going too far is as bad as not going far enough." (**Confucius**)

"A man that is born falls into a dream like a man who falls into the sea." (**Joseph Conrad**)

"Of all the gifts bestowed by nature on human being, heavy laugher must be close to the top." (**Norman Cousins**)

"While we are free to choose our actions, we are not free to choose the consequences of our actions." (**Stephen R. Covey**)

"Success means doing the best we can with what we have. Success is in the doing, not the getting—in the trying, not the triumph." (**Wynn Davis**)

"The past is not dead; it is the sum of the factors operating in the present. The present is the past rolled up into a moment for action; the past is the present unraveled in history for our understanding." (**Will Durant**)

"Logic will get you from A to B. Imagination will take you everywhere." (**Albert Einstein**).

"Your imagination is your preview of life's coming attractions." (**Albert Einstein**)

"Without deep reflection one knows from daily life that one exists for other people." (**Albert Einstein**)

"I never think of the future. It comes soon enough." (**Albert Einstein**)

"Only a life lived for others is a life worthwhile." (**Albert Einstein**)

"It is still the best to concern yourself with eternal, for from them alone flows the spirit that can restore peace and serenity to the world of humans." (**Albert Einstein**)

"It is never too late to be what you might have been" (**George Eliot**)

"To the philosopher, all things are friendly and sacred, all events profitable, all days holy, all men divine." (**Ralph Waldo Emerson**)

"What lies behind us and what lies before us are tiny matters compared to what lies within us." (**Ralph Waldo Emerson**)

"We are always getting ready to live but never living." (**Ralph Waldo Emerson**)

"Those things that hurt, instruct." (**Benjamin Franklin**)

"You can talk about God, and you think about God, but that does not bring God into your presence." (**Joel Goldsmith**)

"An open mind is the beginning of self-discovery and growth. We can't learn anything new until we can admit that we don't already know everything." (**Erwin G. Hall**)

"Pain is inevitable, but misery is optional." (**Tim Hansel**)

"We are closer to God when we are asking questions than when we think we have the answers." (**Rabbi Abraham Joshua Heschel**)

"No matter where you are in life right now, no matter who you are, no matter how old you are—it is never too late to be who you are meant to be." (**Esther & Jerry Hicks**)

"A goal is a dream with a deadline." (**Napoleon Hill**)

"All great truths are simple in final analysis, and easily understood; if they are not, they are not great truths." (**Napoleon Hill**)

"The life so short, the craft so long to learn." (**Hippocrates**)

"The whole thing resolves itself into our mental ability to control our thought. The man who can do this can have what he wants, can do what he wishes and becomes what he wills . . ." (**Ernest Holmes**)

"Experience is not what happens to you; it is what you do with what happens to you." (**Aldous Huxley**)

"Advice is what we ask for when we already know the answer but wish we didn't." (**Erica Jong**)

"We cannot live the afternoon of life according to the programs of life's morning." (**C. G. Jung**)

"If a man is called to be a street sweeper, he should sweep streets even as Michelangelo painted, or Beethoven composed music, or Shakespeare wrote poetry. He should sweep streets so well that all the host of heaven and earth will pause to say, 'Here lived a great street sweeper who did his job well.'" (**Martin Luther King, Jr.**)

"The greatest power that a person possesses is the power to choose." (**J. Martin Kohe**)

"No action, no regret." (**Lao Tzu**)

"In Tao, you should reduce something everyday." (**Lao Tzu**)

"I'm not in this world to live up to your expectations, and you're not in this world to live up to mine!" (**Bruce Lee**)

"Work like you don't need the money, love like you've never been hurt, and dance like no one is watching." (**Randall G. Leighton**)

"And in the end, it's not the years in your life that count. It's the life in your years." (**Abraham Lincoln**)

"In truth, the only difference between those who have failed and those who have succeeded lies in the difference of their habits." (**Og Mandino**)

"The truth never becomes clear as long as we assume that each one of us, individually, is the center of the universe." (**Thomas Merton**)

"Your living is determined not so much by what life brings to you as by the attitude you bring to life; not so much by what happens to you as by the way your mind looks at what happens." (**John Homer Miller**)

"The mind is its own place, and in itself, can make heaven of Hell, and a hell of Heaven." (**John Milton**)

"Don't let the past steal your present." (**Cherralea Morgan**)

"Life is a series of problems. Do we want to moan about them to solve them?" (**M. Scott Peck**)

"Blessed is he who expects nothing, for he shall never be disappointed." (**Alexander Pope**)

"Take care of your body. It's the only place you have to live." (**Jim Rohn**)

"Your life does not get better by chance, it gets better by change." (**Jim Rohn**)

"Do what you can, with what you have, where you are." (**Theodore Roosevelt**)

"Be who you are and say what you feel because those who mind don't matter and those who matter don't mind." (**Dr. Seuss**)

"Do what you love and the money will follow." (**Marsha Sinetar**)

"I am more intelligent than others simply because I know that I am ignorant." (**Socrates**)

"An unexamined life is not worth living." (**Socrates**)

"To be what we are, and to become what we are capable of becoming, is the only end of life." (**Robert Louis Stevenson**)

"It is only when we have the courage to face things exactly as they are, without any self-deception or illusion that a light will develop out of events by which the path to success may be recognized." (**The I-Ching**)

"Those who don't read the news are uninformed. . . . but those who do are misinformed." (**Mark Twain**)

No man or woman really knows what perfect love is until they have been married a quarter of a century." (**Mark Twain**)

"If you don't mind, it doesn't matter." (**Mark Twain**)

"The Sage does not talk, the Talented Ones talk, and the stupid ones argue." (**Kung Tingan**)

"An egg today is better than a hen tomorrow." (**author unknown**)

"There's no great answer to everything. There's only a developing process of which we are a part." **(Jeanette Winterson)**

APPENDIX E

ABOUT THE AUTHOR

About Stephen Lau

http://www.stephencmlau.com

His Publications

http://www.booksbystephenlau.com

His Websites

Chinese Natural Healing
http://www.chinesenaturalhealing.com

Daily Tao Wisdom
http://www.daily-tao-wisdom.com

Healthy and Wisdom Tips
http://www.health-and-wisdom-tips.com

Wisdom in Living
http://www.wisdominliving.com

Wisdom from Books
http://www.wisdom-from-books.com

His Contact
stephencmlau@gmail.com